2/13 for

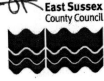

**East Sussex
County Council**

Please return or renew this item
by the last date shown. You may
return items to any East Sussex
Library. You may renew books
by telephone or the internet.

0345 60 80 195   for renewals

0345 60 80 196   for enquiries

**Library and Information Services
eastsussex.gov.uk/libraries**

REMEDIES
& NATURAL CURES

ROTATION
PLAN

D0184929

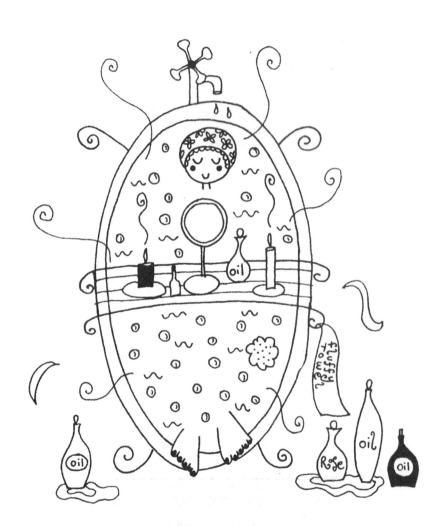

1001
HOME
REMEDIES
&NATURAL CURES

From your kitchen and garden

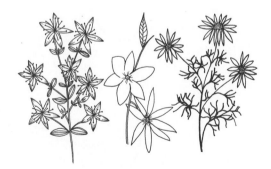

Esme Floyd

CARLTON
BOOKS

THIS IS A CARLTON BOOK

Text, design and illustrations
copyright © Carlton Books Limited 2010

This edition published in 2013 by
Carlton Books Limited
20 Mortimer Street
London W1T 3JW

10 9 8 7 6 5 4 3 2 1

A CIP catalogue record for this book is available from
the British Library.

ISBN 978 1 78097 253 4

Printed in China

Senior Executive Editor: Lisa Dyer
Managing Art Director: Lucy Coley
Design: Barbara Zuñiga
Production: Janette Burgin
Illustrations: Carol Morley

The advice in this book is general in nature, not
specific to individuals or their particular circumstances.
Any plant substance, whether used as a medicine or
a food, externally or internally, can cause an allergic
reaction in some people. Do not try self-diagnosis or
attempt self-treatment for serious or long-term problems
without consulting a medical professional or qualified
practitioner. Do not use herbal preparations or essential
oils without prior consultation with a medical professional
if you are pregnant, taking any form of medication or if
you suffer from sensitive skin. Always seek medical advice
if symptoms persist.

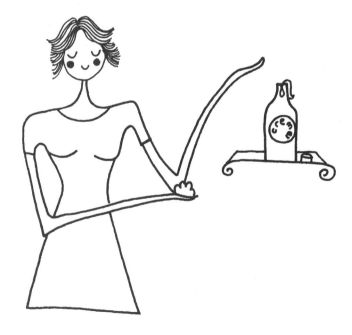

CONTENTS

introduction   6

first aid   12

general ailments   30

internal health   68

musculoskeletal & skin problems 98

bodycare   132

family health   160

lifestyle issues   184

index   222

INTRODUCTION

Remember when your Grandma picked fresh feverfew from her garden to help calm your headaches, dripped clove oil onto your aching tooth or took down her jars of home-made, sweet-smelling creams to keep your sunburn from stinging? Since ancient times, home remedies have been passed down through generations, helping entire families to harness the power of nature to help their bodies heal themselves and stay happy and healthy.

As a child, I used to watch my mother stuffing jars with oil and St John's wort flowers, then we'd watch as the summer sun slowly turned it from yellow to a deep, chestnut brown. She'd use it on cuts, grazes, bruises, bites and stings to help our skin heal, and ever since then I've been intrigued by how, whatever the health problem, nature always seems to provide its own remedy.

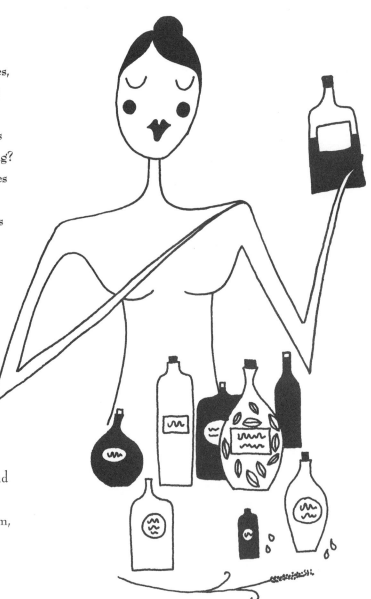

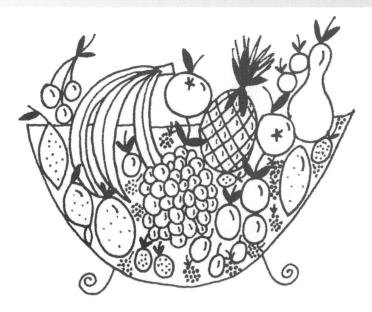

With the busy pace of modern life, it's all too easy to forget about the healing power of nature, but this book brings it together in an easy-to-read reference guide, helping you make the most of the natural products you've already got in your kitchen cupboards or growing in your garden. Although many hi-tech pharmaceuticals have their basis in natural products, home remedies don't take the place of modern medicine, which is why you should always consult your doctor before embarking on any self treatment. Nature's remedies can be used to help your body find the natural strength for a wide range of health issues – fighting infection, aiding good sleep, lessening the effects of colds and flu, beating digestive disorders and even battling depression – and you'll find them all within the pages of this book.

With the pace of life getting ever faster, and medicines ever more complicated and expensive, there's never been a better time to get back to nature and give your body what it deserves – a dose of good, old-fashioned natural healing.

As you peruse the pages of this book, you'll see the same homemade heroes returning again and again, so to help you start out on the path to being a home-remedy expert, here are the top 10 household ingredients and plants you'll need …

Top 10 Plants to Grow at Home

All these homegrown healers can be cultivated in your garden, outdoor pots or windowsill.

1 ALOE (*Aloe vera*) – Ideal for any kind of skin complaint or inflammation.

2 BASIL (*Ocimum basilicum*) – The basis of many relaxing and healing remedies.

3 CAMOMILE (*Anthemis nobilis*) – Calming, relaxing and stress relieving; great for use in infusions.

4 CAYENNE PEPPER (*Capsicum annuum*) – Used in a range of remedies to warm, heal and ward off infections.

5 ECHINACEA (*Echinacea angustifolia, Echinacea purpurea*) – The ultimate immune booster.

6 EUCALYPTUS (*Eucalyptus globulus*) – One of nature's greatest healers and a powerful antiseptic.

7 GARLIC (*Allium sativum*) – Your very own antibacterial, antiviral warrior.

8 GINGER (*Zingiber officinale*) – Almost all remedies for colds and flu need ginger, and it's great for infections, gut problems and other ailments too.

9 LAVENDER (*Lavandula angustifolia*) – Relaxing, calming and a great general healer, as well as an antiseptic.

10 PEPPERMINT (*Mentha piperita*) – Great for digestive problems and reducing stress.

Top 10 Cupboard Essentials

Keep these storecupboard staples well stocked to ensure you always have the right ingredients to create your home remedies.

1 ALMOND OIL – The best carrier oil as it's light and simple to combine with essential oils.

2 APPLE CIDER VINEGAR – The ultimate all-round hero for home remedies, keep it well stocked to help heal a vast range of complaints.

3 BICARBONATE OF SODA (BAKING SODA) – Buy in bulk as it's great for skin problems and many other home remedies, too.

4 EPSOM SALTS – The best choice for aches, pains and other body ailments.

5 HONEY – Helps fight skin and gut problems and a whole range of infections. Manuka honey is a powerful antibacterial, although it doesn't taste as good.

6 LEMONS – Lemon juice is a rich source of antioxidants and vitamins. Fresh is best, but use limes or oranges if you prefer the taste.

7 MUSTARD – A great, warming healer, the smooth, yellow variety is best.

8 OATS – Oats are ideal for treating skin complaints as well as digestive problems. Unrolled are the best choice.

9 SALT – Choose sea or rock salt for the most potent antibacterial and healing effects.

10 TEA TREE – Essential oil of tea tree is a must for any home remedy as it has incredible infection-fighting powers.

Harvesting Plants

Plant's therapeutic properties can be affected by when they are harvested, so pick them on a dry day when they are fully mature as their active ingredients will be more concentrated. If drying the plant, do so away from bright sunlight in an airy, dry, warm place. Herbs take about six days to dry completely and should be brittle to the touch. When fully dry, crumble and discard the stems. Store in clean, dry, dark glass containers with airtight lids. Most will keep for 12 to 18 months.

Flowers should be dried as flower heads or, as in the case of lavender, by hanging from the stem. Seeds should be harvested when almost ripe and hung by the stem to dry – the seeds will fall off when ripe. Harvest berries and fruit when they are just ripe and dry on trays. Bark should be harvested in autumn when the sap is falling and never remove all the bark. Break into manageable pieces and dry on trays. For roots, harvest in the autumn when the aerial parts have died down; they can be washed, chopped and then dried for several hours on trays in a low oven.

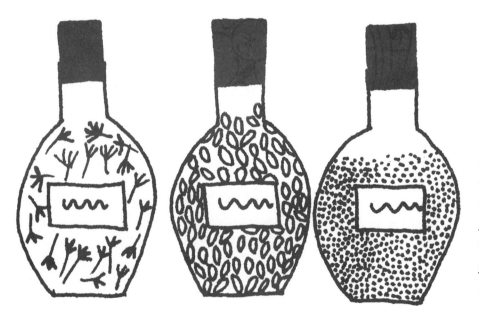

Note: *All plant substances you intend to use should be free of pesticides. Choose organic ingredients if buying from food markets, wash everything thoroughly, and never consume flowers from florists, nurseries, or garden centres.*

Making Remedies

Basic instructions for making the remedies on the following pages are given here, but follow the specific amounts given in individual tips.

TEAS AND INFUSIONS
For herbs, use 1 teaspoon dried or 2 teaspoons fresh chopped herb to 1 cup boiling water. Place the herb in the cup and pour over boiling water. Allow to steep for 10 minutes, then strain.

DECOCTIONS
This method is used for roots, barks, twigs and some berries. Place the ingredients in a saucepan, add cold water and simmer for up to 1 hour until reduced by one third. Standard quantities are 30 g (1 oz) dried ingredient, or 60 g (2 oz) fresh, to 750 ml (1½ pints) water, which reduces to 500 ml (1 pint). Then strain and store in a cool place.

MAKING A COMPRESS
A compress can be administered either hot or cold, and is made by soaking of a cloth pad, bandage or face cloth in an infused solution, such as a tea, tincture or decoction. Be sure to wring the cloth to squeeze out any excess liquid, then hold against the affected area. Repeat when the compress dries.

MAKING A POULTICE
With this method the ingredient is applied directly to the affected area, generally as the hot leaves of herbs or plants. First boil the fresh chopped herb in enough water to cover and squeeze out any extra liquid. If using a dried or powdered ingredient, mix with enough water to form a paste. Then smooth a little olive oil on the skin first to prevent sticking. Apply the poultice warm to the skin, and bind with a gauze bandage or cotton strips to hold in place.

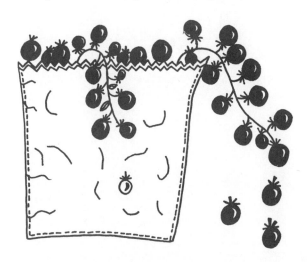

BASIC ESSENTIALS

1 ALWAYS ARNICA

For hundreds of years, the arnica plant (*Arnica montana*) has been used in homeopathic medicine. The blossoms contain sesquiterpene lactones, which are known to reduce inflammation and decrease pain. Apply a topical cream or ointment of the herb on bruises and anywhere the skin is not broken to reduce pain and swelling, and help your skin heal more quickly. Use a strong liquid as a compress on muscle strains and lower dilutions as an oral medicine to help bruises heal quickly.

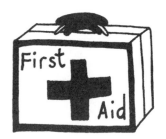

2 LIGHT UP THE LEMON

Not only is lemon a natural antioxidant and high in vitamin C, it has amazing properties as a nontoxic disinfectant and antiseptic, as well as being able to bleach naturally. Always keep fresh lemons at home as the juice can be used to help cure sore throats, soothe sunburn, aid digestion and disinfect wounds.

3 PEAS, PLEASE

For sprains and bruises, a great way to reduce bruising and swelling is to make the area cold, thus reducing blood flow. Even better than shop-bought ice packs are bags of frozen peas, because they mould around the body part to ensure equal distribution of the cold. Place a tea towel next to your skin to prevent ice burn.

4 SAY ALOE TO HEALING

Aloe vera is a first-aid kit essential as it is great for reducing pain and swelling of almost all bites and stings, including jellyfish stings, by simply applying the cooling gel directly to the bite or sting. Easy to grow on a windowsill for constant access, it also helps take the pain and heat out of minor burns and sunburn.

5 VIE FOR VINEGAR

Vinegar is highly versatile. Keep several bottles of cider vinegar in your cupboard, and try infusing them with different herbs so you always have your healing bottles on hand. Thyme and rosemary vinegars make good solutions to soothe bites and stings, while rose vinegar is useful for skin problems.

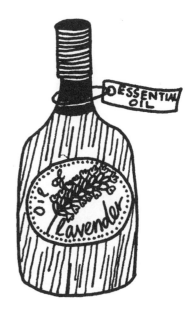

6 LOVE LAVENDER

Lavender oil has highly antiseptic and astringent qualities, and because it's one of the few essential oils that can be applied directly to the skin it's good for the pain relief of headaches, bites, stings and other injuries. It's also great for burns and grazes, where it promotes strong healing and fights infection.

7 TIME FOR TEA TREE

Tea tree oil contains high levels of terpenoids, which are both antifungal and antiseptic, making them a great choice as an ointment where skin is broken to prevent infection and reduce swelling and soreness.

8 YELL FOR YARROW

Yarrow (*Achillea millefolium*) is antiseptic, anti-inflammatory and coagulant, and aids in the healing process for burns, cuts, ulcers and inflamed skin. The leaves can be used as a poultice simply by applying them direct to the skin, or make into a tea.

9 MAKE AN OINTMENT

One of the best ointments you can make for your first aid kit is from St John's wort. Simply cram St John's wort flowers into a large bottle or jar and fill up with good-quality extra-virgin olive oil. Leave in the sunshine every day for three weeks until the mixture turns a reddish brown colour, then store out of the sunlight and use whenever necessary to calm skin reactions to bites, stings, burns, scratches and bruises.

10 GO ON A WITCH HUNT

Witch hazel is a great choice for a first aid box as it is extremely astringent as well as anti-inflammatory, and it stops bleeding as well, which means it's a good choice for cuts, grazes and stings. Keep it in the fridge for maximum cooling relief.

11 BEE PREPARED WITH SALVE

Make up a salve of your favourite healing ingredients by slow-cooking olive oil with essential oils or powders, then strain into a clean glass jar and stir in some beeswax to make a customized salve. Try your own combination of tea tree, mustard and eucalyptus or lavender.

INSECT BITES & STINGS

12 SOOTHE SORES WITH TOMATO

A great way to soothe sore insect bites and stings is to dab on tomato juice. It helps draw out the sting and reduce redness and swelling around the wound. Alternatively, hold a slice of tomato over the area.

13 LIGHTEN PAIN WITH LAVENDER

Lavender not only has relaxing properties, it also helps as an anti-bacterial agent and antiseptic. Mix up your own lavender oil with a few drops of essential oil in a carrier oil such as almond or olive and apply directly to the bite or sting.

14 BAKE THE STING AWAY

Add a teaspoon of bicarbonate of soda (baking soda) to a glass of cold water and stir well. Dip a paper towel or clean cloth in the mixture and place on the bite until it doesn't feel cold any more. Repeat with a fresh towel or different part of the cloth until the pain lessens. Alternatively, make a paste from bicarbonate of soda and water or vinegar and spread on the bite area as a poultice.

15 RUB IT WITH ASPIRIN

If you have just been bitten, you can try moistening the area of the bite or sting and rubbing an aspirin tablet over the top of it for a few minutes to help reduce the pain. The aspirin will help control inflammation. Do not use if you are allergic to aspirin.

16 MASH A PAPAYA POULTICE

Mashed papaya has two important effects when it comes to helping with insect bites and stings – it acts as a natural anti-inflammatory, stopping redness and swelling, and it contains enzymes which act as natural analgesics, reducing pain. Mash fresh papaya and apply directly to the wound.

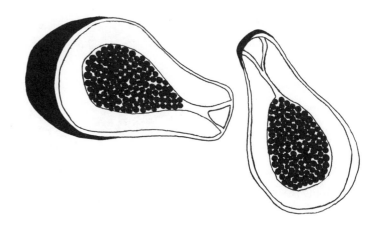

17 DIP IT IN SALT

Dipping an insect bite in hot salty water can help bring some relief – do this as soon as possible after the bite or sting has occurred and leave to soak for a few minutes if possible.

18 OH, FOR ONIONS

If your sting or bite is embedded in your skin, don't try to scoop it out with a sharp implement. Instead, apply a slice of onion onto the area and leave for about 5 minutes, then try to scrape it out with something flat and sharp like a credit card, which won't break the skin.

19 TREAT JELLYFISH STINGS WITH VINEGAR

Steer clear of water for jellyfish stings, as this can actually make the sting worse. Instead, wash immediately in cider vinegar. For the next few days, apply castor oil directly to the sting site twice a day to relieve stinging.

20 HONEY FOR BEE STINGS

Honey is well known for helping to ease the pain of bee stings. Apply a blob of honey directly onto the site of the wound and cover with a dressing, if preferred. Leave for at least 30 minutes to help reduce pain and swelling.

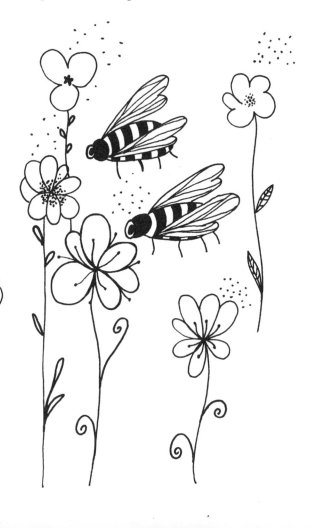

21 ICE PAIN AWAY

You can reduce the pain of insect bites and stings using ice, which constricts the blood vessels and thus reduces swelling. But beware of applying ice directly onto the skin as it can cause burning – instead, wrap in a cloth and dip in water, then massage onto the bite.

22 PICK A POTATO

To help draw out poison from a bee sting or a spider bite, take a slice of raw potato and hold it over the wound for 5 to 10 minutes. You could also use cooked cabbage, which has the same effect. Wrap with a bandage to ensure continued contact.

23 MAKE A TENDERIZED PASTE

If you have powdered meat tenderizer in your cupboard, make a paste of it with petroleum jelly and apply to a sting to help draw out poisons and reduce pain and swelling.

24 WASH AWAY MOZZIE BITES

For mosquito bites, wet a bar of soap and rub directly onto the bite immediately after you've been bitten. The soap helps stop itching and swelling, and works within seconds.

25 SAND AWAY THE STING

A good way to reduce swelling in jellyfish stings is to immediately apply sand to the wound, then try to sit as still as possible for 10 minutes. The sand helps draw out the sting and reduces swelling.

26 USE URINE

If you have the misfortune to be stung by a sea anemone, don't panic. Avoid putting your foot to the ground, which could push the stings in further. Find a comfortable (and private) place, then pass urine into a large bowl and immerse your foot for 10 minutes until all the spines fall out. Wash afterwards with clean, salted water.

27 PICK A PLANTAIN

The broad-leaved plantain weed (*Plantago major*), which grows well in heavy moisture and shade, contains tannins that fight bites and stings by tightening the skin and reduces swelling, itching and pain. For quick relief, grab some plantain leaves, rinse them off, chew to release the juice and then put the chewed piece onto the bite or sting. Hold with gentle pressure until the pain lessens, and repeat, if necessary. Alternatively, rub the leaves together to release the juice and apply to the area.

28 ACTIVATE A CURE

Activated charcoal (available from online stores) can be taken to reduce intestinal toxins and flatulence, but it can also be used for bites and stings. Open up two to three capsules of charcoal, mix with enough water to make a paste and apply to the affected area. After 30 minutes, gently wash the paste off with a wet cloth.

29 GET GARLICKY

Biting insects choose their prey by smell alone and if they don't like the smell of you, they'll steer clear. Eating lots of fresh garlic can help make your skin smell inhospitable to the little critters and they'll move on to tastier morsels, leaving you bite-free.

30 MAKE YOURS A G&T

It is widely thought that the relatively high amounts of quinine in tonic water can help repel mosquitoes and other biting insects. Drink tonic before an evening out and add a slice of lemon too, as that is another smell mozzies don't like.

31 SOOTHE WITH LEMON BALM

The juice extracted from lemon balm leaves may be applied directly to stings and can also be used for cold sores and toothache.

PLANT STINGS

32 CALL FOR CALAMINE

Calamine lotion is the number one treatment for plant stings, especially those that cause inflammation, such as poison ivy. A useful alternative if you don't have any handy is toothpaste, which has the same cooling, drying powers.

33 RUB AWAY THE RASH

A poison ivy rash is the result of the oils from the plant coming into contact with the skin and creating a burn. If you've been exposed to poison ivy, wash your skin with surgical spirit (rubbing alcohol) and then water before the rash has time to appear. Make sure you don't use a cloth, though, which could spread the oil around. Instead, dab or splash the skin.

34 DOCK IT

The next time you suffer a sting from a stinging nettle, look around at ground level to see if you can find nature's cure – a dock leaf (the broad-leafed *Rumex obtusifolius* usually grows near the common nettle, *Urtica dioica*). Simply crush and roll the leaf between your fingers to release the juices and rub directly onto the wound.

35 SPRAY THE STING

If you have a spray can of antiperspirant in your bathroom, you can use it to help cool and calm your skin before rashes like poison ivy appear. Simply spray as directed over exposed skin, but test an area first to ensure you don't exacerbate the rash. Alternatively use water with a few drops of tea tree oil added.

SPRAINS & BRUISES

36 CUP YOUR COFFEE

Caffeine is thought to aid healing. Before you bandage your sprain, slip a tablespoon of black coffee grounds into the bandage, or alternatively soak the inner layer of your bandage in espresso for a similar cure.

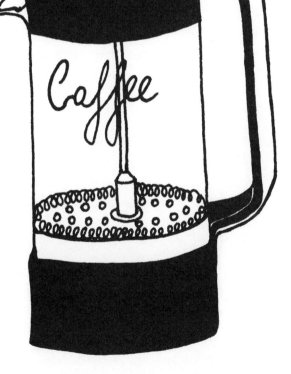

37 GET EGGY

For sprains on wrists and ankles, smear olive oil around the sprain and apply a whisked egg yolk – which is thought to help relieve pain and reduce swelling. Wrap in cotton wool and bandage immediately. Try not to put weight on the affected area, then wash off after one to two days and re-apply until the pain recedes.

38 RUB ON SOME MENTHOL

As soon as you sustain an injury, rub some menthol essential oil onto the site to prevent bruising coming out later that day or the next. Menthol constricts blood flow, which lessens the severity of bruising.

39 MAKE THE BRUISE DISAPPEAR

Mix up some aloe vera and drinking alcohol (tequila, whisky and vodka work best) and apply directly to the bruise to help it disappear quickly.

40 JUST ADD SEASONING

Salt and vinegar can help reduce the pain and swelling of bumps and bruises. Apply the vinegar first with a clean cotton pad, then sprinkle on some salt and rub gently to encourage the bruise to heal more quickly.

41 MAKE A COMFREY POULTICE

Comfrey works as a healing agent due to allantoin – a substance that speeds the production of new cells and aids healing. Grind fresh leaves in a pestle and mortar with enough water to form a paste. Heat in a saucepan over a low heat, stirring constantly, then remove from the heat and cool slightly. Apply to the bruise or sprain and wrap with a bandage to secure.

42 MASSAGE IN MARJORAM

Marjoram is a great essential oil for bruises as it helps reduce pain and swelling. Simply add a few drops of marjoram essential oil to a carrier oil and massage gently into the bruise.

43 WASH WITH VINEGAR

After washing your bruise in the bath or shower, dab on a liquid which is half vinegar and half warm water. Allow to evaporate and repeat three times to help the bruise heal more quickly.

44 GET EGG-STATIC

If you want to help bruises heal more quickly, break an egg into a bowl, whisk up quickly and use a soft brush to baste your bruise. The proteins in the egg are believed to help the skin regenerate more easily and quickly.

MINOR CUTS & GRAZES

45 EARN YOUR BREAD

Applying a slice of bread to a cut can help stop bleeding. Simply hold a piece of fresh bread (either wholewheat or white is fine) over the cut, apply mild pressure and wait for the bleeding to stop.

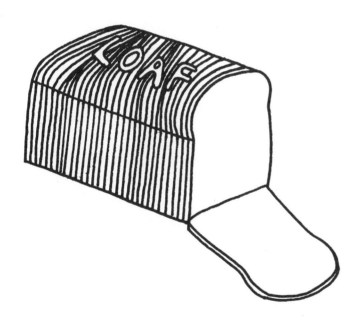

46 SPRINKLE SUGAR ON IT

One of the best ways to help minor cuts heal quickly is to sprinkle a small amount of sugar on the wound and then bandage. Leave for several hours, then wash with clean water.

47 A NATURAL ANTISEPTIC

Marigold is ideal for cleansing an infected cut or graze. Soak the neat or diluted tincture on cotton wool and dab onto the cleaned cut. This may sting, but it is powerfully antiseptic. Washing a cut in strained marigold tea is also effective.

48 HAVE A CUPPA

If you have a cut that won't stop bleeding easily, apply a used, cooled tea bag onto the area. It will also alleviate pain and redness. Tea has a high amount of vitamin K (potassium), which is a natural coagulant, or blood thickener.

49 SPICE IT UP

If you have a cut and you want to stop the bleeding rapidly, sprinkle some turmeric powder on the area. The turmeric will help stop the bleeding and the spice also has anti-inflammatory properties, so will speed healing.

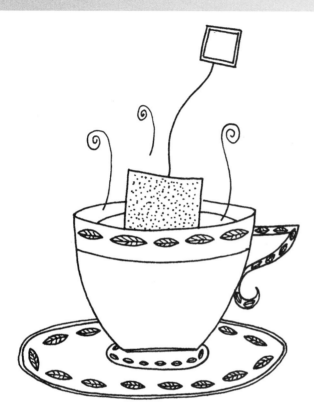

50 CHOOSE A CAMOMILE WASH

Next time you suffer a cut, instead of washing with clean water, brew yourself a camomile tea instead. Pour a little boiling water onto a camomile tea bag, then leave to steep for a few minutes. Remove the bag and top up to halfway with cold water. Use the camomile liquid to wash your wound to reduce swelling.

51 USE GARLIC FOR SPEEDY HEALING

The powerful compound allicyn, which is found in garlic in high levels, is thought to help speed up the healing process, so applying raw crushed garlic or garlic juice to the wound can help.

52 BANDAGE WITH GINGER

If you have suffered a cut, wash the wound well with sterile saline water, sprinkle on ground ginger and bandage as usual. You can also mix ground ginger with enough water to form a paste and apply. The ginger will help reduce pain and swelling, and help prevent infection.

53 YES FOR YARROW

Common yarrow (*Achillea millefolium*) contains isovaleric acid, salicylic acid, asparagin, sterols, flavonoids, bitters, tannins and coumarins and has a long history as a healing herb used topically for wounds and abrasions. To help stem bleeding quickly, sprinkle the powdered dried herb over cuts or grazes.

54 PREVENT SCARS WITH COMFREY

Rub comfrey ointment into the damaged area as soon as possible. It will also help reduce pain and swelling. Do not use on broken skin.

55 ANOINT WITH TEA TREE

Prepare a home-made ointment for grazes with tea tree oil (make sure it's 100%), calendula and comfrey, and apply directly to the affected area to help reduce pain and swelling and help your skin heal more easily.

56 KEEP YOUR EYE ON IODINE

Iodine is widely used in the medical profession for helping to clean wounds and there's no reason why you shouldn't use it at home as well. Simply apply a few drops onto the cut immediately after sustaining it and repeat several times in the first 24 hours.

57 BE A GOOD CHAP

If you suffer a paper cut, it can be difficult to get them to heal as you use your hands so much. Use chapstick to help close up the wound and lessen your chances of infection. Repeat morning and night for best effects, and keep clean.

58 TREAT WITH AN ALCOHOL RUB

If you suffer a small cut, you can help keep it clean and speed up healing by rubbing on some alcohol. Surgical spirit (rubbing alcohol) is best, but anything you can find in your drinks cabinet will do – the higher the alcohol content, the better.

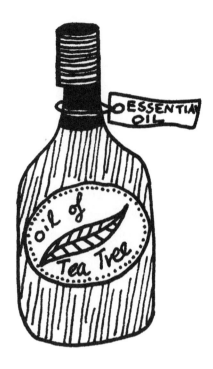

59 BE FRANK WITH FRANKINCENSE

First, clean your graze thoroughly with a bowl of warm water in which you have added 7 to 10 drops of frankincense essential oil (avoid dipping the same cloth – use cotton wool instead and discard after one dip and wipe). When it's thoroughly clean, add 1 or 2 drops of the oil onto the graze and repeat twice a day. This also works with lavender oil, if you prefer that smell.

MINOR BURNS

60 PULP THE PAPAYA

Papaya is great for burns because it has the enzymes papain and chymopapain, making healing quicker and more efficient. After washing with cold water, apply pulped papaya from the fridge directly to the area.

61 EGGS ELEVEN

After cooling the wound with cold water, apply a raw egg to the site of the wound – the egg helps take away excess heat and adds proteins that the skin needs for healing.

62 CHOP AN ONION

This is a good way to help burns heal, particularly in reducing the formation of blisters. Finely chop or mince raw onion, apply to the burn as a poultice and wrap with a clean cloth. Alternatively soak a cold cloth in onion juice and apply as a compress.

63 GET MINTY FRESH

For small burns like those on hands and fingers from cooking, an application of toothpaste can help stop blisters forming and prevent infection. Simply smear toothpaste gently onto cleaned skin.

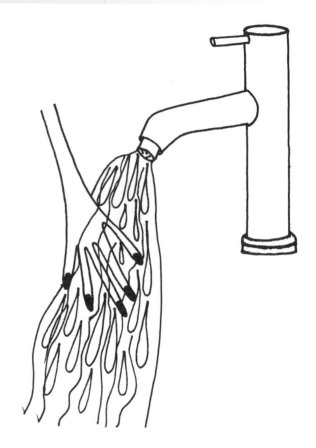

64 KEEP IT COOL

The most important thing if you suffer a minor burn is to keep the area cool – it is the heat of the burn that does most damage to the skin, so reducing the temperature is key. Use cold water rather than ice, which can burn or shock the skin, and apply running water wherever possible to keep it cool.

65 HAVE A HONEY SALVE

To prevent blisters and to help avoid infection as the burn heals, apply honey directly onto the burnt area of skin (after washing with cool water). Honey contains enzymes which help kill bacteria, so it's a great choice to encourage healing.

66 SUCK ON SUGAR

If you burn your tongue on hot food or drink, immediately sprinkle granulated sugar on it – the sugar takes in the heat and helps prevent the tongue from feeling scorched for too long.

67 REMOVE THE BURN WITH A POTATO

Because potatoes are so good at holding heat, they are a great anti-burn remedy to keep in your fridge. To draw heat from burns, simply take a raw potato from the fridge, grind to a paste and apply directly to the burn site.

68 MAKE IT BETTER WITH BUTTER

Once you have cooled the burn site by holding under cold running water or soaking in cold water, dry carefully (patting only to avoid skin trauma) and smother the burn in butter. This re-oils the skin and prevents drying and blistering, which can lead to pain and scarring.

69 CUT SOME ALOE LEAVES

Aloe vera gel is a great choice for burns, but the leaves work even better. Cut the leaves in half lengthways and apply directly, juice side down, to the site of the burn. Leave for 10 minutes, preferably with an ice pack on top to keep skin cool as well.

NOSEBLEEDS

70 GET A COLD NOSE

If you suffer from nosebleeds, it's worth keeping a cloth or flannel in the fridge so the minute your nosebleed starts, you can hold the cold cloth to the bridge of the nose and/or forehead. This constricts blood vessels and stops bleeding.

71 USE LEMON TO STOP BLEEDING

Place a few drops of lemon juice into the nostril that is bleeding. Lemon is a natural antiseptic and can help stem bleeding by constricting blood vessels.

72 APPLY VINEGAR TO CONSTRICT BLOOD

Dip a cotton ball or clean cloth in apple cider vinegar and apply this to the bleeding nose until the blood stops. The vinegar helps the blood to congeal and clot.

73 DAB WITH GOLDENSEAL

Add 1 teaspoon goldenseal or echinacea tincture to 500 ml (1 pint) water and heat up this mixture in a saucepan or microwave until it boils. Remove from the heat and allow to cool. When cool, use some if it to coat the inside of the nostrils.

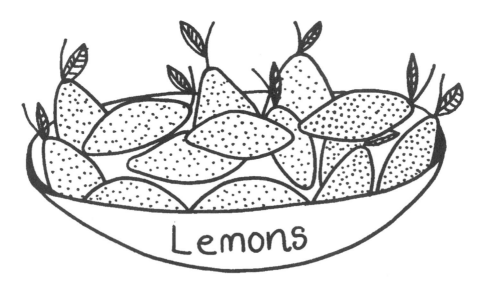

Lemons

SPLINTERS

74 GET STUCK IN

A great way to get splinters out of a wound is to use children's craft glue. Put it over the site of the splinter, allow to dry and simply pull out – it will bring the splinter with it. Alternatively, try sticking tape securely to the splinter site and pulling away slowly to take out the offending article.

75 SOAK IT AWAY

Soaking the affected body part in Epsom salts can work because it helps draw out any impurities. Sprinkle Epsom salts into a bowl of warm water and soak for 10 minutes or until the splinter drops out.

76 SLIP IT OUT WITH SLIPPERY ELM

A poultice made from the powder of slippery elm (available from health food stores) will coax the splinter out of the skin, and will also help heal the damaged tissue. Marshmallow root can be substituted for slippery elm.

77 PLAN A PLANTAIN POULTICE

Draw out the splinter with a salve made from the leaves of the plantain. Alternatively, blend the crushed fresh leaf with a little water to make a paste and apply to the area, securing with a gauze bandage.

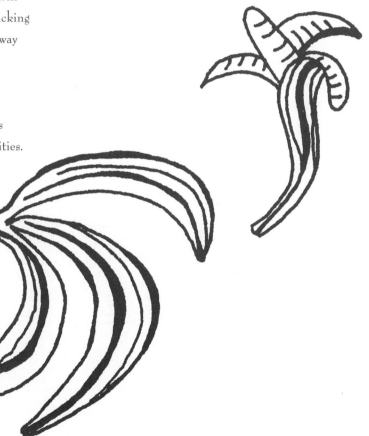

SUNBURN

78 DIP IN VINEGAR

Add a cup of cider or white vinegar to a bath of cool water and sit in it for as long as you feel comfortable. This will help reduce the skin's redness and soreness. Pat dry carefully and apply a moisturizer.

79 WASH WITH STRONG TEA

It might sound like a strange idea but making yourself a strong pot of tea and allowing it to cool with the bags still in it, then using the liquid as a wash, can help reduce the pain of sunburn. The natural tannins in the tea are thought to lower blood flow, reducing swelling and soreness.

80 SOW YOUR OATS

Fill a sock or stocking with oatmeal and hang it under the tap as you run a bath so the water flows through it. Remove the bag before you bathe, and try to stay in the water for at least 10 minutes. This is also a good remedy for poison ivy.

81 DOCTOR YOUR MOISTURIZER

To a plain moisturizer, add a few drops of aloe and tea tree oil, then use liberally over areas affected by sunburn. If you suffer a lot, you can even make up a bottle of this homemade concoction and keep by your bed to apply when you feel sore or tight.

82 BAKE YOUR BODY

Instead of bubble bath, sprinkle baking soda (about a cup) into your cool bath and rather than drying yourself off afterwards, allow your skin to dry naturally, which will naturally cool it down.

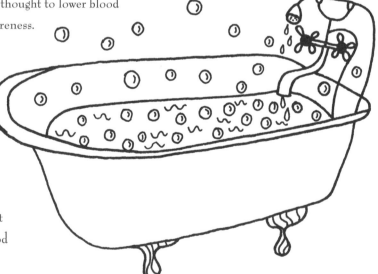

CRAMPS

83 MAKE A HOT DRINK

Cramps are most often caused by heavy exercise, cold, illness, menstruation or a strain. As soon as you feel the cramp coming on, drink a cup of hot tea or coffee to give yourself a dose of heat and caffeine. Try to sit and relax for a few minutes while it takes effect, then continue as normal. The warmth will increase your blood flow and relax your muscles.

84 GET PICKLED

Next time you suffer a cramp, drain off a few tablespoons of pickle juice and drink immediately to help the muscle repair with no lasting damage. The juice contains water, salt, calcium chloride and vinegar (acetic acid), and is thought to act like an isotonic beverage.

85 BATHE IN FLOWERS

If you suffer from cramps at night, add a few camomile tea bags to your evening bath. This will aid relaxation and could also help prevent muscles cramping in the early hours as the flower has antispasmodic and anti-inflammatory properties.

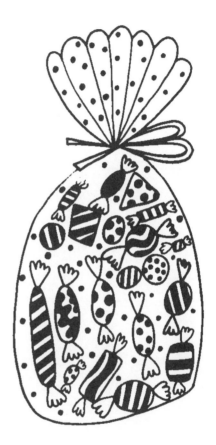

86 TOOT SWEETS

Muscles can cram because they lack fuel so stave off your muscle cramps, especially if they follow exercise, with a lollipop sweet or a handful of jellybeans or jelly babies, which contain sugar and carbohydrates.

ANAEMIA

87 WAKE UP SWEET

Every morning, drink up a cup of lemon and honey mixed with hot water. This will help boost your iron absorption levels throughout the day and make anaemia less likely.

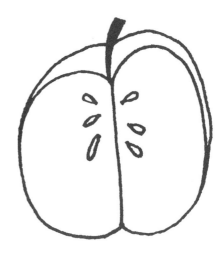

88 AN APPLE A DAY

Eating a couple of apples every day could help your body maintain iron levels by boosting vitamin C intake, which is essential for iron absorption. If you don't like apples, two or three fresh or dried figs or apricots could also help.

89 GET WITH THE BEET

Juice a beetroot and add a handful of crushed or juiced mint leaves (a drink rich in minerals like potassium as well as B vitamins) to help give your body's iron storage system a boost and reduce anaemia.

90 DICE SOME DANDELION

Dandelion is rich in all the nutrients your body needs to keep its iron levels high, such as manganese. If you tend towards anaemia, eat some dandelion leaves with your salad to boost iron absorption.

FEVER

91 BOIL AWAY FEVERS

For a natural cure for fevers, boil up some holy basil with powdered or crushed cardamom seeds and mix with some fresh milk. Add sugar to taste and drink twice a day to reduce fevers.

92 HAVE A TODDY

Drink a cup of tea with a dash of rum or cognac added to it to help bring down your fever. Note this is for adults only!

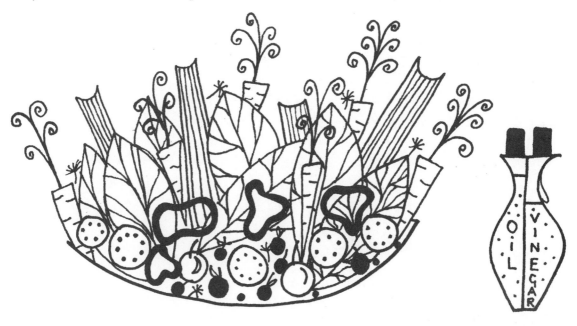

93 ROT OUT FEVER

Horseradish root is thought to help the body's temperature system to regulate itself. Grind or chop fresh horseradish root into a cup of boiling water, steep for 5 minutes, then drain and drink. If you don't like horseradish, use 1 teaspoon mustard seeds instead.

94 SAY SORREL

Wood sorrel has high levels of vitamins and minerals which can help healing, and is also thought to reduce fevers and chills. Boil up the leaves in water, drain and drink with honey to taste.

95 SOAK YOUR SOCKS

It might sound strange, but feet are key to body temperature, so many home remedies for fever involve the feet. Soak your socks in vinegar for 5 minutes before putting them on to help reduce your fever.

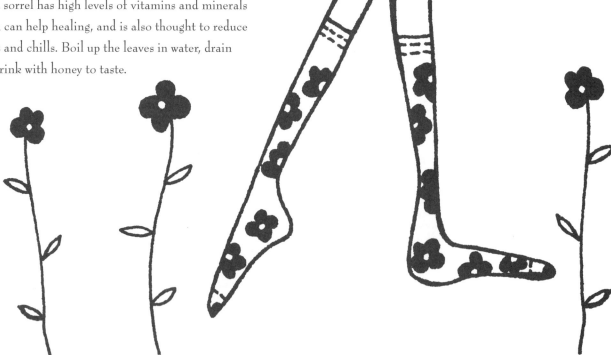

96 COOL DOWN YOUR FEET

Try rubbing your feet with surgical spirit (rubbing alcohol) or dipping your socks in alcohol and putting them on. This cools down your feet, which helps your body regulate its temperature.

97 MAKE A BANDAGE

Grind up some barley and mix it with ground sesame (a pestle and mortar is great for this), then cook it gently in milk until it thickens. Use this to soak a bandage or flannel and apply to the forehead to reduce fever.

98 ASK FOR ARRACK

The South Asian alcoholic drink arrack is thought to help reduce fevers, either rubbed onto the feet or chest area. Alternatively make a mixture with ½ cup arrack and ½ cup water and apply to the forehead with a flannel or washcloth.

99 GO STEEP

Thyme has antiseptic properties, camomile reduces inflammation and linden promotes sweating, so try steeping 1 teaspoon of each dried herb in 1 cup boiling water for 5 minutes. Strain and drink warm several times a day.

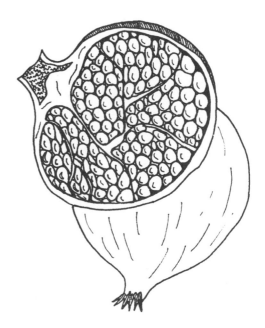

100 EAT POMEGRANATES

Eating fruit and drinking water is thought to be a good way to naturally reduce body fevers. Pomegranates, carrots, apples and grapes are all good choices.

101 GET PEPPERY

Mix up a handful (about 8) shredded basil leaves with 3 or 4 black peppercorns, then chew on them together. Alternatively, make yourself a 'fever busting' meal by sprinkling these on top of a green leafy salad.

102 MAKE BASIL TEA

Basil has very strong antipyretic (fever-reducing) properties, so make up a batch of the tea with the fresh or dried leaves if you have a fever. Drink a cup every few hours throughout the day.

103 INFUSE YOUR TEA

Instead of making your normal cup of tea with milk, make the an anti-fever drink. Make a cup of tea as normal but add in a pinch cinnamon powder, 2 large cardamom seeds and a pinch ginger powder or some fresh ginger. Allow to steep for 5 to 10 minutes, and remove the cardamom before drinking.

104 BE A POTATO HEAD

Cut some slices of potato, then lie down on a bed and place the potato slices where you feel they will help most to bring down your fever – head, chest, stomach and eyes are all good places to start.

105 DRESS YOUR FEET

Crush 2 large cloves garlic and mix with 2 to 3 tablespoons warmed olive oil. Apply the mixture to the sole of each foot and wrap in plastic. Wear overnight or until the fever disappears.

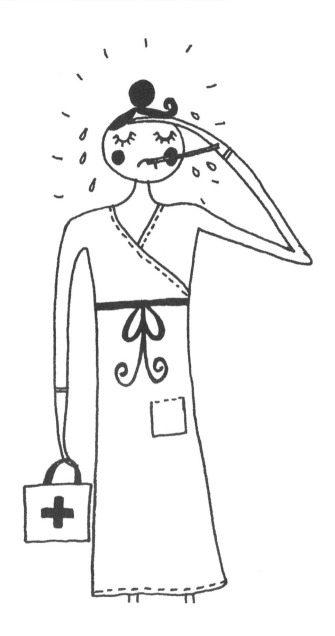

34

106 KNOW YOUR ONIONS

Peel a large onion and slice it in half, then attach each half to the sole of each foot and relax with your feet elevated for an hour.

107 EAT YOUR FRUIT

Fruit and vegetables will treat fevers as they fortify the body's immune system without taxing the digestion. Orange and grapefruit are great choices, while apricot juice mixed with honey is another good fever fighter.

108 SOAK SOME SAFFRON

Brew up an anti-fever remedy by soaking 1 teaspoon saffron in 50 ml (¼ cup) boiling water, then leave to steep for about 10 minutes before straining. Take a teaspoon of the mixture every hour to help reduce fever.

109 RAISIN THE STAKES

Crush 10 g (⅓ oz) raisins with 10 g (⅓ oz) fresh sliced ginger and mix with 200 ml (7 fl oz) water. Let stand for an hour, then boil to reduce until one-quarter of the mixture is left. Drink once or twice a day until fever reduces. The mixture can be stored for two to three days in the fridge.

110 TAKE TAMARIND

In Ayurvedic medicine, tamarind leaves have been used in tea for reducing fever. Prepare a cold drink by mixing a pinch of turmeric powder with 2 fresh tamarind leaves in 125 ml (4 fl oz) cold water. Drink to help reduce fever and repeat twice a day.

111 LEAN ON LINDEN

Linden tea is a great anti-fever infusion as it can induce sweating due to the flavonoids in the linden blossoms, which in turn helps bring the body temperature down. Steep 1 tablespoon of the fresh flowers in 1 cup of boiling water for 10 minutes before straining. Drink regularly until the fever reduces. The drink will induce perspiration, which releases heat from the body.

112 BARKING MAD

Willow bark (*Salix alba*) is rich in natural chemical compounds called salicyclates (from which aspirin is made) and is thought to be nature's very own fever medication. Steep 1 teaspoon powdered willow bark in ½ cup of water for 10 minutes. Drink ½ cup no more than twice a day. Black elder flower (*Sambucus nigra*) is a good alternative, especially for people who can't tolerate aspirin.

SORE THROAT

113 BE SAGE

Make a tea infusion by steeping 3 to 4 fresh sage leaves in hot water for 5 to 10 minutes with a pinch of cayenne pepper. Allow to cool and strain before using the mixture to gargle. If you like, you can also drink the tea.

114 RED SAGE WITH HONEY OR VINEGAR

Red sage is a little-known garden herb but it's great for sore throats. Infuse 1 teaspoon powdered red sage in 1 cup boiling water. Cover and leave for 10 minutes, then divide the mixture in half. Drink half with honey and add a dash of vinegar to the rest for use as a gargle.

115 INFUSE YOUR HONEY WITH ONION

Add ½ peeled onion to a jar of honey, close tightly and leave for at least three days. Take a teaspoon of the onion honey every few hours to reduce the severity of a sore throat.

116 CHOOSE CINNAMON AND MILK

Cinnamon is a great cure for sore throats. Stir ¼ to ½ ground cinnamon into a glass of hot milk or boiling water, then add a pinch of cayenne pepper. Drink to reduce pain and discomfort in your throat.

117 SOOTHE WITH SPICE

Make a homemade sore-throat medicine by mixing together 1 teaspoon cider vinegar, a pinch cayenne pepper, the juice of ½ small lemon and 1 teaspoon honey. Add to 1 cup of hot water and stir well to combine. Allow to cool, then drink. Repeat three times a day.

118 MAKE IT A MANGO GARGLE

Mango is anti-asthmatic, antiseptic, antiviral and an expectorant. Ideally use the juice extracted from mango bark (*Mangifera indica*), mixing 10 ml (⅓ fl oz) of the juice with 125 ml (4 fl oz) water and using as a gargle to soothe the throat. Alternatively, you can infuse mango extract or dried mango fruit (readily available in supermarkets) in boiling water, then allow to cool and use as a gargle.

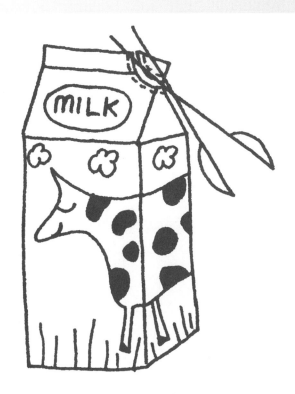

119 A MILK SOLUTION

Sore throats are often caused by rawness, which is why some traditional remedies contain milk to soothe and coat the raw throat. Gently heat 125 ml (4 fl oz) milk with 1 tablespoon butter and 1 tablespoon honey until combined. Drink slowly to coat the throat. If you don't like milk or can't tolerate dairy products, use a cup of hot grapefruit juice with a spoonful of honey dissolved into it.

120 GARGLE WITH SALT

Make a simple homemade painkilling gargle with warm water and a little salt. Mix well and use to gargle deep into your throat several times a day.

121 CALM WITH CAMOMILE

Make yourself some camomile tea either by using a shop-bought tea bag or preferably with dried camomile blossoms – infusing 1 or 2 teaspoons dried camomile in 500 ml (1 pint) boiling water. The herb soothes scratchy membranes in the throat and will help stop the irritation.

122 REDUCE PAIN WITH GINGER

Ginger is anti-inflammatory, antiviral and a painkiller, so it's great for sore throats. Make up a batch of ginger tea using freshly grated ginger root in boiling water (around 1 tablespoon per cup) and allow to infuse for about 10 minutes. Drink a cup at regular intervals throughout the day.

123 CRAM IN THE CRANBERRIES

Cranberry juice is good for easing sore throats – just gargle and drink. Try to use it as cold as possible, which can help reduce swelling.

124 PICK SOME PARSLEY

Parsley's medicinal properties help treat winter ailments such as coughs, colds and sore throats. Make a tea using fresh flat-leaf parsley leaves and gargle or drink it to soothe your sore throat. Aim for 3 to 4 cups daily while the throat is still sore.

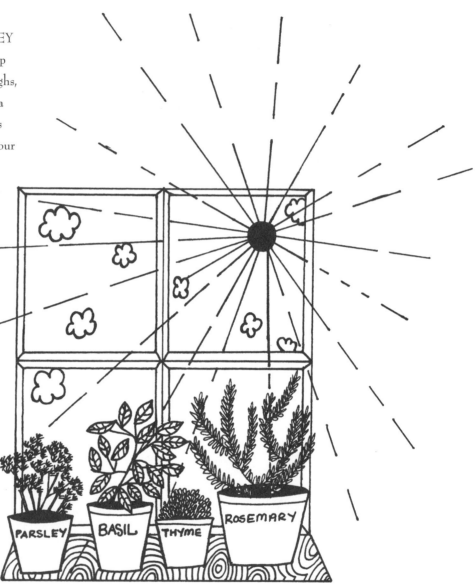

125 DRINK CHILLI, CINNAMON AND GINGER TEA

Instead of making yourself a cup of tea the next time you have a sore throat, make an infusion with ¼ to ½ teaspoon chopped red chilli pepper, ½ teaspoon ground cinnamon and 1 teaspoon fresh chopped ginger root in a cup of hot water. Sweeten with honey or maple syrup and add lemon or lime juice or slices for flavour. Drink as soon as you notice a sore throat appearing.

126 FLAVOUR YOUR TEA WITH MEDICINE

Boost the medicinal effects of an ordinary cup of tea by adding a sore throat lozenge (the stronger sweets containing menthol are the best types to choose) and some honey to sweeten. Take twice a day.

127 SOOTHE PAIN WITH MARJORAM

To help lessen the severity of a sore throat, drink marjoram tea made with either the fresh or dried herb. Marjoram has natural anti-inflammatory properties so is good at soothing pain. Sweeten with honey or sugar if preferred.

128 PICK UP A PINEAPPLE

To help sore throats, especially if you are losing your voice, eat canned crushed pineapple – the acidity of the pineapple helps to reduce swelling and to clear out mucus and bacteria from the throat surface.

129 MUNCH ON MUSTARD

Mustard is thought to have great healing properties, so eating it when your throat is sore could help to reduce pain and swelling. Eat a teaspoon of mustard on its own twice a day. The yellow, smooth variety is best, but any type will help.

130 MIX A VINEGAR GARGLE

A good way to help heal your sore throat is to add 1 tablespoon cider vinegar to 1 cup of warm water. Mix well and use as a gargle. Gargle with each mouthful for 10 to 15 seconds, then swallow. Repeat until the cup is finished.

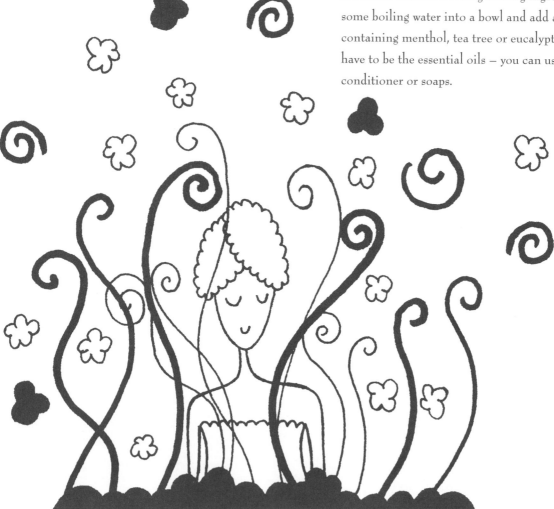

131 INHALE AWAY PAIN

One of the things that can really help a sore throat is a steam inhalation using healing ingredients. Pour some boiling water into a bowl and add anything containing menthol, tea tree or eucalyptus. It doesn't have to be the essential oils – you can use shampoo, conditioner or soaps.

SINUS PROBLEMS

132 CONCOCT A VINEGAR AND HONEY DECONGESTIVE

Fill up a jar with honey, then vinegar to the proportions of ¾ vinegar to ¼ honey. With the lid tightly screwed on, shake well. Store in a dark cupboard. To aid decongestion, take a spoonful or mix with hot water to make a drink.

133 DO AN OIL PULL

First thing in the morning, before brushing teeth, eating or drinking, take 1 tablespoon of sesame or sunflower oil into your mouth and swish for 10 minutes. Do not swallow or gargle and do it as slowly as possible – the oil should be white and foamy when you spit it out. Follow by drinking at least 250 ml (8 fl oz) of water. This is an old Indian remedy designed to remove bacteria from the mouth.

134 GRAB A GRAPEFRUIT

If you have some grapefruit seed extract, simply sniffing it is a great way to help cure sinus problems. For a similar effect, try eating fresh grapefruit, drinking a hot grapefruit infusion or grating grapefruit peel into hot water to inhale.

135 SEEDS OF CHANGE

Mix mustard seed powder with just enough water to form a paste. Dab a tiny amount inside the nostrils and breathe in and out normally to help clear congestion.

136 TURN ON THE HEAT

Eating a diet rich in chilli (especially jalapeño peppers) and low in dairy products is reported to help clear sinus congestion. Try this for a few days at the onset of blocked sinuses.

137 HAVE A CRUSHED GRAPE

Ripe grape juice (red or white) is a good anti-congestion remedy. Take it in place of milky drinks either hot or cold, according to your preference. Or juice up your own grapes for a concentrated dose.

138 BREATHE IN A EUCALYPTUS INHALATION

Eucalyptus oil works by thinning the mucus in the respiratory tract and relieving congestion. Drop a few drops of eucalyptus or tea tree oil into some boiling water and inhale the steam through your nose for 20 minutes Adding oats can help if your nose feels raw and irritated.

139 TOP WITH A BASIL–CLOVE PASTE

Many home remedies involve spreading a topical paste onto your skin to help relieve internal blockages. For sinus relief, mash together 5 to 6 basil leaves, ½ teaspoon each ground cloves and ginger to form a paste. Apply over the painful sinus area – on either side of the nose and the forehead. Avoid getting too near the eyes and don't apply if you have sensitive or reactive skin. Leave for 5 minutes before rinsing off.

140 WATCH FOR WASABI

Wasabi (the pale green hot horseradish sauce served as an accompaniment to Japanese food) has a very powerful sinus-clearing action because one of its main constituents promotes mucus flow, and it is also good at flushing out the eyes by causing them to water. Incorporate in your diet to alleviate sinus congestion.

COMMON COLDS

141 EAT FISH AND SEAFOOD

Zinc is thought to cut the length of colds by several days so if you want to get better more quickly, make sure you're getting enough by choosing fish and seafood, which have high levels. Red meat, beans and nuts are also good sources of zinc.

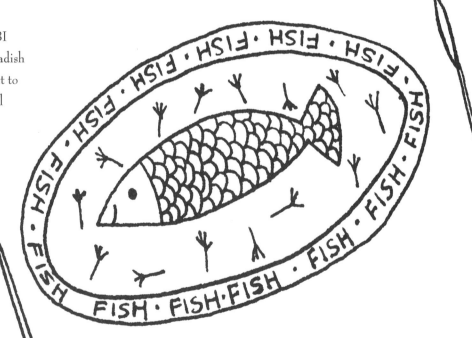

142 SOUP IT UP

It's an old favourite, but that's because it really does work. Make up a batch of chicken soup at the first sign of a cold. It's important to include the old-fashioned ingredients of onions, sage and garlic in your recipe as they are thought to be linked to the healing properties. Ingest a bowl or cup twice a day while you have a cold.

143 TAKE GINGER FOR MUCUS BUILD-UP

Fresh ginger is a great warming root to use to fight congestion caused by colds and it helps break down mucus. Make a tea by grating a 2 to 3 cm (¾ to 1 in) piece fresh ginger root into a cup. Pour over boiling water and leave to stand for 30 minutes. Add honey or maple syrup to taste.

144 DRINK A LEMON AND HONEY TODDY

It's a cure that's as old as the hills, but a honey and lemon toddy does work against colds. Squeeze ½ fresh lemon into a cup, then add 1 teaspoon honey and a dash of brandy. Pour over hot water. Drink slowly, inhaling the steam. If you like, add a pinch of crushed garlic or powdered ginger.

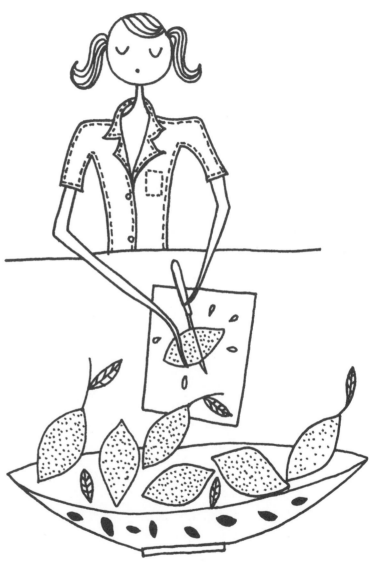

145 PUT A PINCH OF PEPPER IN YOUR SOUP

Make yourself some warming chicken or vegetable soup (but avoid adding too much milk or cream, which can encourage mucus production). Add a few pinches of cayenne pepper – the two types of heat combine to help your cold melt away.

146 EASE WITH ECHINACEA AND VITAMIN C

If you feel a cold coming on, immediately reach for echinacea, which is known to help boost the immune system. Combining a few drops of the tincture with high levels of vitamin C from fruit or vegetable juice can enhance the effects.

147 FIX COLDS WITH FENUGREEK

A pungent herb that can help reduce mucus and lessen fever, fenugreek (*Trigonella foenum-graecum*) is used for both its seeds and leaves. Make a tea by steeping 1 teaspoon whole fenugreek seeds in 1 cup boiling water for 10 minutes, then straining. Drink twice a day to help relieve congestion. A common ingredient for curries, the seeds can be harvested from the plant and dried in early autumn, or purchased at a supermarket or health food store.

148 GET GARLICKY

Garlic soup is one of the oldest remedies for beating common colds. Boil 3 to 4 cloves garlic in 1 cup of water, strain and drink every day while you have a cold. Or make up a drink with ½ teaspoon garlic oil and 1 teaspoon onion juice in warm water, which serves the same purpose.

149 FIND COMFORT WITH COMFREY

In a saucepan combine several chopped comfrey leaves and ½ cup fresh elderberries (you can substitute cranberries or redcurrants). Mix in 1 cup each honey and water and simmer for 30 minutes. Drink as a tea to ease discomfort and reduce mucus. The solution can be stored in an airtight container in the fridge for one or two days. Reheat thoroughly to use.

150 DRINK CINNAMON AND GINGER MILK

At the onset of a cold, scald a cup of milk and add ½ teaspoon each ground cinnamon and ground ginger. Stir well. The hot drink will help warm your system, boost immunity and prevent symptoms from worsening. You can also substitute turmeric powder for the cinnamon and ginger.

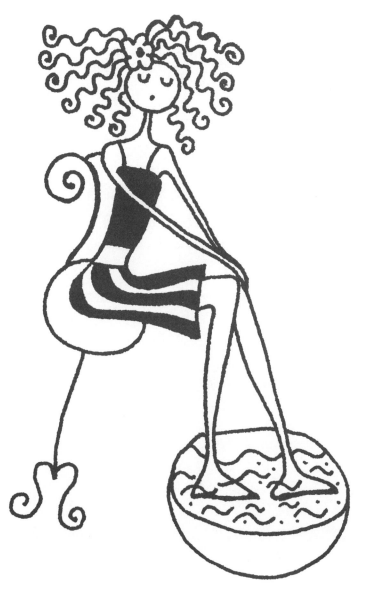

151 BATHE YOUR FEET IN MUSTARD

Strange as it may sound, foot baths have been known to help reduce sold and fever symptoms. Pour 3 litres (5 pints) of water into a footbath with 2 tablespoons dried mustard powder and soak your feet for 20 minutes. Do not use if you are diabetic, have poor circulation or if any area is inflamed or has an open wound.

152 MAKE A FRUIT SOUP

This homemade medicine will help stave off the worst cold symptoms. Mix 1 tablespoon chopped ginger root, 2 tablespoons honey and a handful of raisins with 500 ml (1 pint) of water and simmer for an hour. Cool, strain and refrigerate overnight. The next morning, add the juice of 2 lemons and 1 orange. Mix well and drink a glass twice a day.

153 CHEW A CURE

Chewing fresh parsley is a good cold cure as it helps to freshen breath and reduce congestion by thinning the mucus build-up in the nose and throat. Simply wash and chew fresh leaves for several minutes.

HEADACHES

154 PASTE YOUR HEAD

Sandalwood (*Santalum album*) is known for its relaxing and cooling properties, and is used in Ayurvedic medicine to relieve fever and burns. If your headache is caused by tension then a sandalwood powder paste could help reduce pain and stress. Combine pure sandalwood powder (available from herbal stores) with enough water to form a paste and apply over the forehead. Allow to dry, then rub and wash off. Ground cloves can be used substituted for the sandalwood.

155 HONEY YOUR HEAD

To reduce the severity of a headache, stir a teaspoon of honey into a glass of water and drink at room temperature.

156 APPLY A SPICE POULTICE

Grind together equal amounts of almond, clove and cinnamon. Add a little warm water to make a paste, then apply to the forehead and jaw. Leave for 5 to 10 minutes until dry, then rinse off. These spices will help reduce the severity of tension headaches. Alternatively mix a little ground cloves into cinnamon oil instead (available from herbal stores).

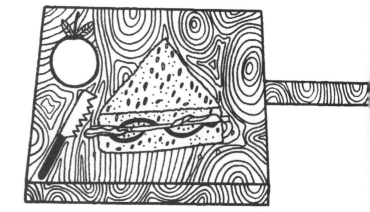

157 EAT A FEVERFEW SANDWICH.

Feverfew is a herb that has long been associated with reducing the pain of headaches. Make up a sandwich with feverfew in white or wholewheat bread and eat with a glass of water to help reduce pain.

158 WILL THE WILLOW

White willow (*Salix alba*) is the number one herbal remedy for headaches. It's a natural cousin of aspirin, which can help block pain signals, so reducing headache and other pain. A tea can be prepared from 2 grams dried willow tree bark boiled in 200 ml (7 fl oz) of water for about 10 minutes, before straining and drinking.

159 WISH FOR WATERMELON

Watermelon juice is cooling and hydrating and is a traditional Ayurvedic medicine for headache reduction. The fresh juice is best, and you should aim for two glasses a day while your headache lasts.

160 MASSAGE IT AWAY

Use a simple carrier oil, such as sesame, almond or mustard oil, to massage your scalp to reduce headache pain. To aid relaxation, add cinnamon or rosemary to the oil first.

161 BREATHE IN MUSTARD

A mustard poultice can help alleviate headache pain. Mix ½ teaspoon mustard powder with 3 teaspoons water, then use a cotton bud to spread the mixture inside the nostrils to reduce headache pain.

162 ROLL ON THE ROSEMARY

Rosemary oil is thought to be a good headache beater as it aids relaxation in the muscles of the forehead. Use rosemary oil (or make your own with olive oil infused with fresh rosemary) and massage into the forehead, jaw and behind the ears. Leave for 10 to 15 minutes before washing off.

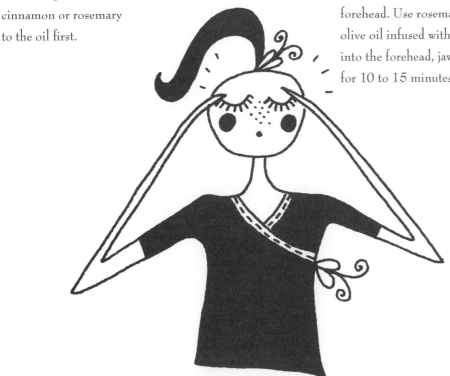

163 EAT AN APPLE WITH SALT

If you suffer from headaches regularly, make sure you include apple in your diet as it is thought to have the right levels of antioxidants and vitamins to reduce the chances of suffering pain and complications. Cut and sprinkle on a little salt before eating it first thing in the morning.

164 ICE IT AWAY

Applying an ice pack to the painful area of your head could help you reduce the pain of your headache – use frozen peas or a proper ice pack, and wrap in a teatowel or t-shirt to avoid 'cold burn' on your skin.

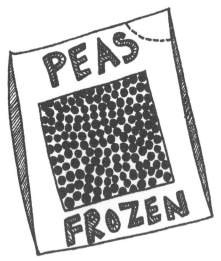

165 RELIEVE MUSCLE PAIN WITH MUSTARD

To relax the muscles of the neck and shoulders, which may be contributing to your headache pain, dip a cloth or small towel in a mixture of warm water and mustard powder. Drape the cloth around your neck and relax for 5 to 10 minutes.

166 USE A ROSEMARY INHALATION

Rosemary works well as an inhalation as it has natural analgesic (painkilling) properties and also helps you relax. Pour boiling water over a few sprigs of rosemary and inhale the steam deeply.

167 GET HOT AND COLD

Headaches can often respond to hot and cold temperatures – soak two face cloths in bowls of water, one hot and one cold, and alternate applying them to your forehead and/or neck for a minute at a time. Do this for 5 to 10 minutes.

168 HENNA YOUR HEADACHE

Henna flowers are thought to have anti-pain properties. Rub the flowers in vinegar and apply over the forehead for quick relief. Aim to leave them there for 5 to 10 minutes before wiping clean.

169 MAKE A MARIGOLD MASSAGE OIL

Pound a handful of fresh marigold flowers with 1 tablespoon olive oil in a pestle and mortar. Mix with a little more oil in a jar and cover tightly. Store for several days. Use the oil to massage painful areas of your head and neck to bring relief.

170 EASE YOUR HEAD WITH HERBS

Make a herbal sachet by mixing together equal amounts of dried lavender, marjoram, rose petals and rose leaf. Add about half the amount of cloves and dried rosemary. Sew the herbs into a cotton or muslin sachet and keep beneath your pillow to help reduce headaches at night.

171 BATHE YOUR FEET

It might seem strange, but bathing your feet in a hot footbath is thought to 'draw' the pain away from your headache. Do this every night for 10 minutes before bed and your headaches should start to reduce.

172 BAG A BANANA

Bananas are high in potassium which can help muscle headaches – eat a banana as your headache starts to appear, but try to limit yourself to 1 large or 2 small bananas a day.

173 CHEW A BUNCH OF BASIL

Take a handful of basil leaves and chew them up together until they turn to a mush, then discard. Once this is done, your headaches should have diminished or disappeared.

174 LIGHTEN UP WITH LAVENDER

If your headaches are caused by stress, you can help reduce the pain with calming and relaxing lavender. Put 3 drops lavender oil onto a sugar cube and suck slowly.

175 RING THE ROSES

Rose essential oil is excellent for reducing headache and inducing relaxation. Add a few drops to a warm bath and sprinkle in some fresh rose petals. Alternatively, add a few drops of rose essential oil to a cold compress and apply to the forehead for 10 to 15 minutes.

176 RUB YOUR WRIST WITH ROSES

Make up your own refreshing rose rub by covering a small glass jar of red rose petals with pure (medicinal) alcohol and leave to stand uncovered in the sun for a day or two. Strain and use as a rub on the wrists and temples to relieve headache.

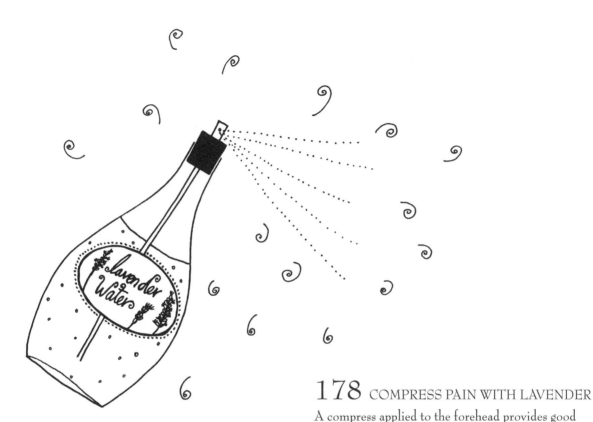

177 ALMONDS AND MILK

If you are prone to headaches, every day eat
6 almonds alongside a glass of hot milk in your
diet at breakfast or bedtime. Add honey or black
pepper to the milk if you prefer.

178 COMPRESS PAIN WITH LAVENDER

A compress applied to the forehead provides good
relief for headaches, especially if you make your own
dressing. Mix 500 ml (1 pint) surgical spirit (rubbing
alcohol) with 1 teaspoon ground cinnamon, 1 grated
nutmeg, 1 teaspoon dried cicely, 2 teaspoons dried
lavender and 2 tablespoons lavender water. Seal and
let stand for two weeks, then strain and cover. To use,
soak the compress in the lavender solution and apply
to the forehead for 10 to 15 minutes.

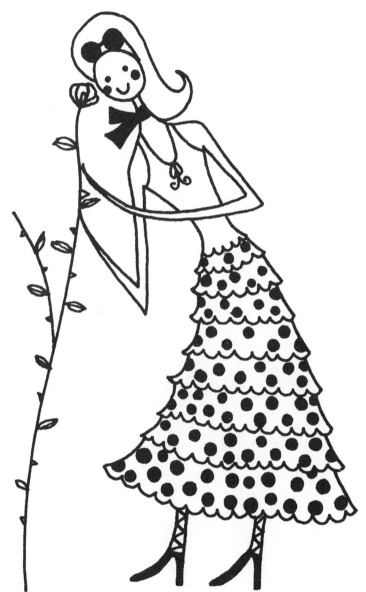

179 ROSE PETAL VINEGAR

Make a batch of rose petal vinegar by filling a wide-necked jar with scented rose petals and slowly pour over warmed white malt vinegar. Seal and leave on a windowsill for two to three weeks, agitating daily. Use as a medicine, dressing, inhalation or rub to soothe headache pain. You can use the same process to make lavender or watercress vinegar.

180 MIX UP A PERSONAL OIL

The best massage oil for a headache is one you can easily make yourself (and preferably get someone else to massage it into your head and neck). Using almond oil as a carrier oil, add a few drops of essential oil – peppermint, rosemary, clove, aniseed, wintergreen, marigold or any mixture of these, depending on what makes you feel most relaxed when you smell it. Experiment to find your ideal mixture and write it down so you can repeat it.

COUGHS

181 RUB YOUR FEET TO ALLEVIATE A COUGH

Instead of rubbing Vicks VapoRub or a homemade alternative like menthol and eucalyptus on your chest, rub it onto the soles of your feet. Massage for a minute or so, cover with warm socks and go to bed. You'll be amazed at how quickly this remedy works.

182 SUCK A LEMON

A great way to stave off coughs is to cut a lemon and grind black pepper over it, then suck the peppery lemon to reduce coughs and help soothe tickly throats.

183 SYRUP YOUR TEA

Make up a batch of lavender tea and sweeten it with maple syrup. Take a warm cup of the tea two or three times daily to help stop your cough naturally.

184 PEPPER YOUR HONEY

To 1 teaspoon of honey add a pinch of white or black ground pepper and eat, swallowing slowly. Repeat two to three times daily.

185 MAKE AN ONION MEDICINE

Finely slice a red onion – make the slices as thin as possible – and put them in a shallow container. Drizzle over some honey and cover tightly for three to five hours, until the onion has released all its juices. Strain and keep the liquid, then take 2 tablespoons every hour to lessen your cough.

186 REDUCE COUGHS WITH RASPBERRY

Make up some raspberry leaf, raspberry or liquorice tea, as these are all linked to a reduction in coughing. Allow the tea to steep for 5 to 10 minutes before drinking. Be careful not to drink raspberry tea if you are pregnant, though, as it could have deleterious effects.

187 GO GINGERLY

Ginger is excellent for helping to reduce coughs as it has anti-inflammatory effects. Make ginger tea or chew raw peeled ginger root a few times a day to get the full effects.

188 RAISIN THE STAKES

Soak 100 g (3½ oz) raisins in water to cover for 30 minutes, then grind together to make a paste using a pestle and mortar. Add 100 g (3½ oz) sugar or honey and heat until it turns to a gravy-like consistency. Take about 5 teaspoons before bed.

189 BE READY WITH ROOIBOS

Make up a tea with rooibos (red bush) tea and add a few leaves of holy basil and a few drops of aniseed. Drink twice a day to help get rid of dry coughs. The rooibos has potent antioxidant and immune-modulating effects, but you can substitute green tea or regular black tea for the rooibos.

190 MAKE UP A MARJORAM CURE

Place 1 teaspoon dried marjoram – or 1 tablespoon fresh – in a cup and add boiling water. Leave for 5 to 10 minutes, then drink and repeat three to four times a day to reduce the severity of your cough.

191 PASTE IT ON

Make a homemade cough medicine by mixing together 1 teaspoon black pepper, 1 teaspoon fresh chopped ginger root, 2 tablespoons each apple cider vinegar and honey and ½ cup water to make a paste. Take a tablespoon a day to help your cough.

192 ONION AND COMFREY COUGH SYRUP

Make your own cough syrup by baking onions in the oven and extracting the juice, then mix the juice with comfrey tea and honey to create a thickish liquid. Take a tablespoon night and day to help soothe a dry, irritating cough.

193 GET GARGLING

A good, easy way to reduce coughing is to gargle with warm salt water. This reduces the amount of phlegm in the throat, lessening the likelihood of coughing.

194 TIME FOR TURMERIC

Turmeric is a great herb for helping to reduce coughing and it is best taken as an inhalation. Sprinkle 1 teaspoon turmeric into a bowl of boiling water and stir. Then lean over the bowl and breathe in the steam for several minutes.

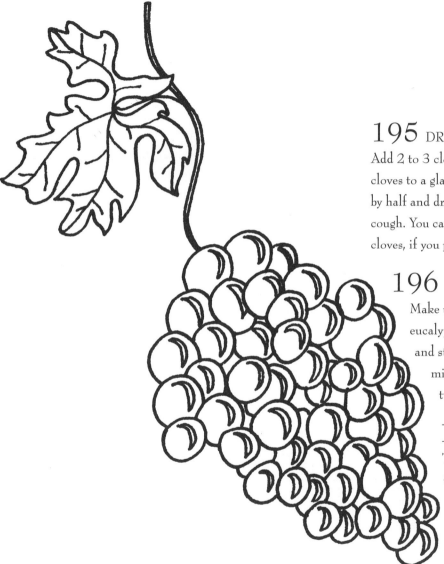

195 DRINK UP A CURE

Add 2 to 3 cloves crushed garlic and 3 ground cloves to a glass of milk. Heat to reduce the amount by half and drink while still warm to lessen the cough. You can substitute oregano instead of the cloves, if you prefer the taste.

196 BREATHE IN EUCALYPTUS TEA

Make up a cough-reducing tea using fresh eucalyptus and mint leaves, slightly crushed and steeped in hot water for 5 to 10 minutes. Add honey to taste and drink twice daily for relief.

197 GET YOUR GRAPES

There's a reason why grapes are the traditional foodie gift for people in hospital – the little bundles of goodness contain chemicals that act as expectorants, helping you shift stubborn mucus on your lungs.

ALLERGIES

198 PASTE AWAY ALLERGIES

Mix 1 teaspoon sandalwood powder (available from herb stores) with enough lime juice to form a paste. Apply to the area affected by the allergy to help calm and soothe the reaction. The poultice will also help reduce itching. After 5 minutes, rinse off with lukewarm water.

199 GO COCO-NUTS

Coconut oil is a great natural moisturizer, and when combined with lemon juice it can be a great way to minimize allergic reaction – simply mix half and half and use as an ointment to calm the area.

200 BE A POPPY

Crush 1 tablespoon poppy seeds in 1 teaspoon water and 1 teaspoon lemon juice. Use the resulting paste to apply to the allergic area to get relief.

201 RUB AWAY ITCHING WITH PAPAYA

If you are suffering an allergy that is causing you to itch, mash up some papaya seeds in a little papaya juice. Use the paste to apply directly to itchy areas to bring relief.

202 MAKE AN ALMOND LEAF POULTICE

Mash up a few almond leaves with a little olive or sunflower oil in a pestle and mortar. Apply the mixture directly to the affected area to bring relief from allergic reactions and calm swelling and itching.

203 C THE DIFFERENCE

High doses of vitamin C can help the body control allergic reactions. Get yours from eating citrus fruits, carrot juice or cucumber juice. Better still, make an anti-allergy juice drink using any fruit or vegetable juice with 5 drops castor oil mixed in (and drunk on an empty stomach).

204 DRINK SOME MINT

Garden mint is a good way to help lessen the severity of allergic reactions, especially to plants. Simply make up some strong mint tea using crushed mint leaves, add sugar or honey to taste, and drink a cup twice a day.

205 CIDER YOUR WATER

To a glass of cold water add 2 tablespoons cider vinegar and mix well. Drink at least once a day to help reduce the allergy.

206 TREAT HIVES WITH COOL MILK

Wet a cloth with cold milk and place it directly on
the affected area for 5 to 10 minutes for relief from
hives and other itchy skin allergies.

207 GO GREEN

Drinking 2 to 4 cups of green tea a day (without
milk) is a good way to help ease allergy as the tea
contains substances thought to reduce swelling.
Sweeten with a little honey if you must, but drinking
it plain and hot is most effective.

208 COMBAT HAYFEVER WITH PEPPERMINT

Peppermint tea is thought to help reduce allergies
like hayfever, which cause congestion. Simply drink
a cup of (preferably fresh) mint tea morning and
evening to reduce symptoms. Peppermint also has
anti-inflammatory and antibacterial properties.

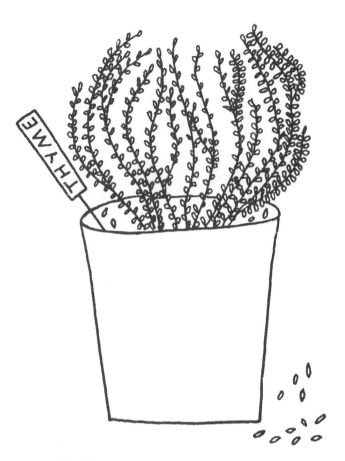

209 A SPOONFUL OF HONEY

Local honey is thought to be able to help against
allergies to airborne allergens like pollen and seeds,
such as hayfever, because it is likely to contain a wide
range of pollens. Choose varieties that have come
from your geographical area.

210 THYME FOR TEA

To help reduce allergic reactions, make a cup of
thyme tea by steeping 1 teaspoon dried thyme (or
1 tablespoon fresh) in 1 cup of hot water for 5
minutes, then straining and drinking. Add honey to
taste, if you prefer, and repeat morning and evening.

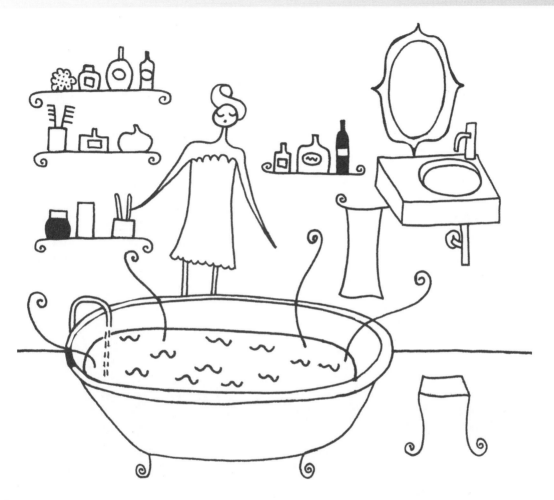

211 BATHE IT AWAY

For skin allergies, pour ½ cup bicarbonate of soda (baking soda) into your bath and soak for around 20 minutes. This should help reduce redness, swelling and itching anywhere on the skin. For hard-to-soak areas like the face, dip a flannel in the mixture and apply to the area for several minutes.

212 USE NETTLES FOR HAYFEVER

If you suffer from hayfever, you can help lessen the effects by preparing yourself a drink of nettle tea twice a day – the plant is thought to have compounds which limit the release of histamine, slowing allergic reactions.

213 ICE IT AWAY

Ice is useful for helping to calm allergic reactions as it can constrict blood flow to the area it is in contact with, thus reducing swelling and itching. For skin reactions, apply directly, but for runny noses or sneezing apply it to the sinuses (at the top of the nose and above the eyebrows).

214 IRRIGATE YOUR NOSE

Nasal irrigation is an effective way of treating nose allergies. You won't look your best during the process, but it will help make your nose less sore and itchy so it's worth a try. Mix 1 cup lukewarm water with ½ teaspoon each salt and bicarbonate of soda (baking soda), then use an ear syringe to gently squirt the mixture up one nostril while holding the other closed. Lower your head over a bowl or sink and gently blow out the water, then repeat the other side and so on until the water is gone.

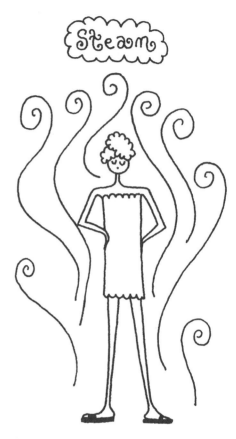

215 GET STEAMY

Breathing in steam helps to reduce pain and inflammation in the nasal passages and the throat, as it soothes on contact. Pour boiling water into a bowl or run the shower on hot and close the bathroom door to create a homemade sauna.

216 GET IT TO A T

Tea tree oil is good for calming allergic reactions, especially if the skin is red and swollen, as it reduces swelling and protects against infection. Apply neat or as a compress to the affected area.

217 BATHE IN BASIL

To help relieve allergies on the skin, try washing the affected area in basil tea (made using fresh basil leaves and hot water, then allowed to cool and strained). Basil is very effective for skin disorders as it kills bacteria and soothes inflammation. Apply the tea as a rinse as often as needed to calm itching skin.

218 STEEP SLICES OF GINGER ROOT

Ginger is a natural antihistamine, which means it reduces the presence of allergens in the blood. Eat yours peeled and sliced raw, or brew a tea with fresh ginger root slices in hot water, adding lemon or honey to taste.

219 SNIFF IT UP

If your nose is the cause of your allergy problems, sniffing a saline solution could help by reducing the amount of allergens in your nasal passage and getting rid of excess mucus. Check with your doctor first before sniffing anything, if you have asthma.

HERPES

220 SAY ALOE TO HEALING

Aloe vera is a great herb to use on cold sores, particularly to help the skin renewal process after they have scabbed over. Squeeze out some juice from the fresh leaves, or use gel or lotion if you prefer.

221 FREEZE IT AWAY

Ice works as an anti-inflammatory agent so it's very useful to reduce sores as they appear. At the first sign of a sore appearing, wrap ice or an ice pack in a thin towel or cloth and apply to the area for 10 minutes.

222 CHOOSE MANUKA OINTMENT

Manuka honey is a great cupboard essential. Made from the pollen of the tea tree, it has fantastic antibacterial and antiviral capacities, so it's great to use as a topical anti-cold sore treatment. Apply a thin layer as an ointment several times a day.

223 BAKE IT AWAY

Baking powder can be used to help clean and dry out sores to prevent infection and reduce severity. Simply dampen a clean cloth or cotton wool ball, dip in the baking powder and apply to the sore.

224 HAVE A CUPPA

Black tea (*Camellia sinensis*) contains very high levels of tannins, which have both an anti-inflammatory and anti-viral effect, so they are great for reducing herpes attacks. Make a cup of black tea and leave it to cool a little. Apply the warm or cooled tea bag to the affected area for 5 minutes and repeat several times a day.

225 GET STARCHY

Cornstarch is a good way to dry out sores to stop them spreading or becoming infected, particularly if they are in the genital area. Simply dust a light coating of cornstarch on the affected area to dry and reduce discomfort.

226 SUPPORT YOUR IMMUNE SYSTEM WITH CASTOR OIL

Boosting your immune system makes you less likely to suffer a herpes attack and a good method is to use a castor oil pack. Soak two thicknesses of face cloth or hand towel in 1 cup castor oil, then lie down and relax with the cloth over your abdomen. Secure with cling film (plastic wrap) and cover with a heating pad. Rest for one hour – this is thought to help boost natural immunity.

227 TREAT RAW AREAS WITH ESSENTIAL OILS

If your skin is left reeling red, raw or inflamed after an outbreak, apply some essential oil (or one mixed with a carrier oil depending on your preference) to the area. Try vitamin E, jojoba, rosehip, calendula or hypericum.

228 DAB ON COLD MILK

Applied cold from the fridge and dabbed onto cold sores or herpes outbreaks with a cotton-wool ball, milk is thought to reduce pain and lessen the severity of outbreaks.

229 HAVE A SALT BATH

If your outbreak is in the genital area, taking an Epsom salts bath could help relieve your itching and tenderness. Pour in as directed and soak for 10 to 15 minutes. Dry carefully afterwards to reduce irritation.

230 STOP OUTBREAKS WITH TEA TREE

Tea tree oil, a natural antiviral agent, is great for killing the virus that lurks in cold sores, helping the sores heal and reducing your chances of passing them on to someone else.

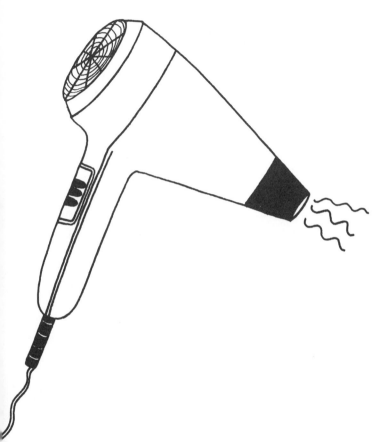

STOMACH BUGS

232 REHYDRATE WITH COLA

Cola or electrolyte sports drinks are a great choice if you've been vomiting and had diarrhoea because they not only rehydrate you but replace lost electrolytes and salts like potassium, sodium and glucose.

233 MAKE AN ELECTROLYTE-REPLACING DRINK

Fill a glass with half fruit juice and half water, then add ½ teaspoon honey and a pinch salt. Drink once or twice a day whenever you feel dehydrated.

234 TAKE TANNINS

Sometimes it's the foods you're eating rather than a virus or bacteria that can cause stomach upset. If this is the case, drinking green or black tea (without milk) can help as the tannins will help to settle sore tummies.

235 FIZZ IT UP

Make up a super-fizzy rehydration drink with a couple teaspoons of sherbert (powdered candy) in 125 ml (4 fl oz) soda, such as cola. Drink in sips or small amounts to settle your stomach.

231 COOL DRY WITH A HAIRDRYER

For genital herpes, use a hairdryer on a 'cool' setting and direct air to the area for a few minutes. This helps dry out the area and reduce inflammation, lessening the chances of infection developing and spreading.

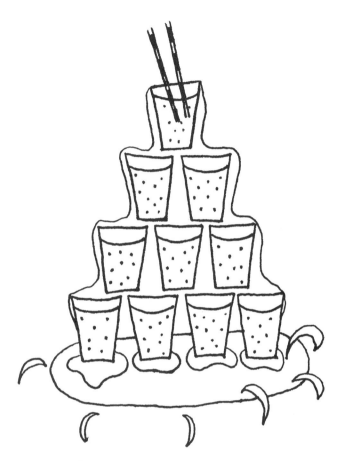

237 CALL FOR CHARCOAL

Charcoal is a great neutralizer, absorbing the contents of your stomach and transporting it to the colon. Mix activated charcoal (available from online stores) with hot water and drink. This is especially useful in the case of accidental poisoning.

238 REPLACE YOUR BACTERIA

As you recover from a stomach bug, make sure you eat 2 to 3 tablespoons live (active culture) yogurt every day to help re-culture your stomach and digestive system with helpful bacteria.

239 COOK YOUR APPLES

Eating slightly cooked apples (preferably sprinkled with a little honey or sugar and some salt) is a good way to reduce stomach pain and swelling because of the high levels of pectin they contain (pectin will help repair the gut lining). Eat half to a whole cooked apple every morning.

236 DRINK UP

The first thing to do if you have a stomach bug or food poisoning is to drink lots of water. If your stomach is too sensitive to keep even this down, raid your fridge and suck on ice cubes instead, which will help rehydrate you without causing nausea.

240 CHEW ON GINGER ROOT

Peel a piece of raw, fresh ginger root and hold it between your teeth. Gently bite down to release a little juice and repeat every few minutes to help reduce nausea and vomiting.

241 MAKE A MUSTARD SANDWICH

For a stomach ache, lightly toast a piece of wholewheat bread, then spread with mustard and eat several mouthfuls. The mustard has a calming effect and the bland toast helps to reintroduce sugars and salts to your body.

242 SHOOTERS STRAIGHT UP

If you can tolerate alcohol, mix up 80 to 90 ml (2½ to 3 fl oz) of clear vodka with 1 teaspoon salt and drink. This helps to alter the stomach lining to make it less receptive to bacteria. For a non-alcoholic alternative, use warm vinegar.

243 BE A BRAT LOVER

To help you recover from stomach bugs, spend two days on the BRAT diet (that is, Bananas, Rice, Apples (lightly cooked) and Toast). This will help your digestive system return to its normal state without strain.

244 MAKE A LEMON REHYDRATOR

A great homemade rehydration salt can be made by mixing the juice of 2 to 3 lemons with 1 teaspoon bicarbonate of soda (baking soda) and a pinch of salt. Drink immediately.

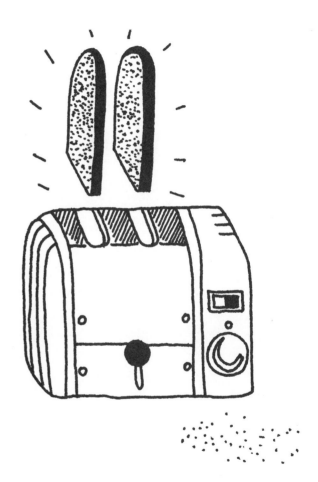

PARASITES

245 CRUNCH A CARROT

If you have worms, changing your breakfast could help remove them naturally. Before taking medication, try eating 2 grated carrots for breakfast instead of your usual cereal or toast until symptoms disappear.

246 FLUSH OUT WORMS

Mix 1 tablespoon papaya juice with 1 teaspoon honey in a glass and fill up another glass with warm milk to which you have added and mixed 1 teaspoon castor oil. Drink the juice, and then the milk, on an empty stomach first thing in the morning to remove worms.

247 PICK A PUMPKIN

Pumpkin seeds are thought to have anti-parasite properties. Peel and grind ripe pumpkin seeds and soak the grinds in warm water for several hours. Strain, and take 2 to 3 tablespoons twice a day to help you become parasite-free. If all this all seems too much, you can simply eat a handful of raw pumpkin seeds a day, but the effect won't be as potent.

248 DE-WORM WITH MINT

Take a handful of fresh spearmint leaves and extract the juice, either using a juicer or by steeping in a small amount of hot water for an hour and straining. Add lemon juice and a pinch rock salt. Drink daily to help remove worms.

249 WAVE A POM-POM

Pomegranate juice is thought to be helpful if you are suffering from stomach worms. Drink a glass of fresh pomegranate juice a day while you have symptoms. This is also believed to help prevent worms infecting you, if taken regularly.

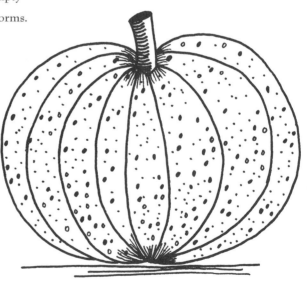

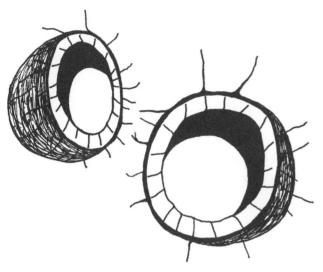

250 GO COCO-NUTS

Eat coconut or coconut milk three to four times a day while you have parasites and they should disappear within a few days. Coconut is thought to make the stomach and bowel unreceptive to worms, flushing them out in the stools.

251 GET PUNGENT

Peel and thinly slice 1 whole head garlic into a small saucepan and add 1 cup milk. Bring to the boil, remove from the heat, cover and refrigerate overnight. In the morning, strain and drink on an empty stomach 30 minutes before you have breakfast. Repeat for a total of three days.

252 BACK TO BLACK

Black walnut (*Juglans nigra*) is a powerful anti-parasitic and the most powerful part is the inner bark of the walnuts themselves. If you buy black walnut, check it is from the bark. Or make your own tea by scraping out the inside of a black walnut shell and using 1 teaspoon inner bark to 1 cup of hot water.

253 CLOVE THE WAY

Cloves also have anti-parasitic qualities. Use the spice to make an infusion by grinding the cloves in a pestle and mortar. Alternatively buy oil of cloves and dissolve 5 to 10 drops in water, then drink to help cleanse your system of parasites.

254 GET FISHY

Fish oils can be used to discourage lice from infesting your hair. Smear fish oil generously on the scalp, rub in, leave for a few hours and wash off.

255 MAKE IT WITH MAYO

Mayonnaise might not seem the obvious anti-parasitic choice, but it's a great anti-lice treatment for hair. Cover the head in mayonnaise, then wrap with cling film (plastic wrap) and leave overnight. Shampoo out in the morning.

256 BATHE IN MILK

If you are suffering from a tapeworm infestation
(the easiest way to diagnose this is that you will be
passing larvae or eggs in a bowel movement) an easy
home remedy is to bathe in milk. Lie as still as you
can for at least 10 minutes and the theory is that the
tapeworm will swim towards the milk, thus expelling
it from your body.

257 GET RID OF LICE WITH ROSEMARY

A great way to get rid of headlice is to drop rosemary
oil onto your hair. Massage into the scalp to repel
headlice as they can't cope with the smell.

258 SUFFOCATE YOUR LICE

Drench your hair in olive oil, cover in cling film
(plastic wrap) or a showercap and leave
for eight hours or overnight. By the end
of that time, all the headlice will have
suffocated and your infestation
will be gone. You could also
use petroleum jelly
or unsalted margarine.

259 DROWN TICKS WITH KEROSENE

Alcohol or kerosene applied to the whole head area of
the tick can cause it to stop embedding itself and seek
somewhere else to live. Be prepared to wait, though; it
could be 10 minutes before anything happens.

260 REMOVE RINGWORM WITH FIG LEAF

To remove ringworm from the skin, break a fig leaf
in half, extract the white sap and rub directly onto
the lesion several times a week. You can also use
black walnut extract or green walnut hulls (crushed
into a pulp) for the same effect.

261 PASTE ON GINGER

Make a paste using 1 tablespoon ground ginger
and 2 to 3 drops echinacea or goldenseal essential
oil. Apply directly to the lesion several times a day
while symptoms last and keep the paste refrigerated
between applications.

262 GO STRAIGHT

Lice can't deal with extremely high temperatures,
so using heat-powered styling tools like hair
straighteners, could help kill any lice you have
in your hair.

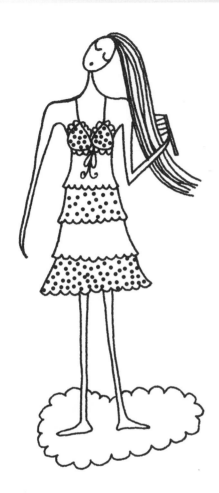

264 PROTECT AGAINST LICE

The most effective home remedy for headlice is to make a preventative oil using 20 drops each of rosemary, tea tree and lavender essential oils in ½ cup olive oil and ¼ cup vinegar. Apply, leave overnight and wash in the morning.

265 CURE WITH LEMON AND GINGER

Take 250 ml (8 oz) lemon juice and add 1 teaspoon grated fresh ginger root. Rub thoroughly into dry hair, concentrating on the areas at the back of the head and behind the ears. Cover with a shower cap and leave overnight, then wash and comb hair in the morning.

266 LIGHT MATCHES FOR TICKS

If you have a tick, don't pull it out of the skin quickly as you might make things worse. Instead, light a match, blow it out and hold it to the abdomen of the tick. As the tick feels the heat, it should draw its head back out of your skin.

267 SPRAY IT OFF

For any parasites that affect your skin, nails or hair, you can make up a generic anti-parasite spray. Place 100 ml (3½ fl oz) apple cider vinegar in a spray bottle and combine with ½ teaspoon each lavender and tea tree essential oils. Spray liberally directly on the affected area several times a day.

263 COMB IT OUT

Whatever home remedy you choose to get rid of lice, make sure you always use a fine-toothed 'nit comb' after the treatment to ensure all the eggs and carcasses have been removed.

ASTHMA & BREATHLESSNESS

268 WARM UP YOUR BANANA

Limit the severity of asthma attacks with a warm banana and a sprinkling of black pepper. Peel a banana, mash or slice it and heat gently. Sprinkle over the pepper, then eat while still warm to gain the best benefits. This is not a cure, simply a tool to lessen the severity of attacks – if you're feeling wheezy, it can help to reduce tightness.

269 TAKE YOUR TURMERIC

Grind an old piece of turmeric (traditionally thought to increase potency) into a powder using a pestle and mortar. Add 1 tablespoon turmeric powder to 2 tablespoons honey and eat daily until symptoms lessen.

270 GET A DOG

There's not a lot of scientific evidence but it's an old myth that having Chihuahuas in your house could lead to fewer asthma symptoms and attacks (unless it's a dog allergy which causes it). Something in the dog's dander is thought to help combat the condition, but it's best to investigate before buying one!

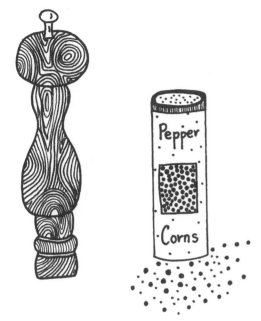

271 CHEW PEPPERCORNS

Every night before going to bed, chew a few black peppercorns. If the taste is too severe for you to handle, mix them with some basil or holy basil (tulsi) leaves, which are also beneficial.

272 SNIFF SOME HONEY

For immediate relief from wheeziness caused by asthma, hold a jar of (open) fragrant honey under the nose. Honey is thought to be one of the best anti-asthma cures, and even smelling it can help make breathing easier.

273 DRINK FROM A COPPER CUP

Before you go to bed, put a glass-worth of drinking water in a copper vessel. In the morning, drink the water before eating anything. You will absorb small amounts of the mineral copper, which is thought to reducing congestion and tightness.

274 MULL OVER SAGE

Make a homemade tea by infusing 1 tablespoon each dried mullein (*Verbascum thapsus*) and dried sage in 1 cup of hot water for 5 minutes, then strain and drink. Use mullein flowers if you prefer a sweeter taste. An old herbal favourite for respiratory problems, mullien is a great remedy for asthma, bronchitis and cough, and the herb grows widely in the US and Europe.

275 DILUTE YOUR JUICE

Instead of water, drink a glass of diluted lemon juice with every meal. This will help combat asthma in the long term by boosting vitamin C levels and acidity.

276 MASSAGE AWAY ASTHMA

Massaging your chest area with mustard oil and camphor is a good way to help reduce breathlessness as it both increases circulation and helps dilate airways and reduce congestion.

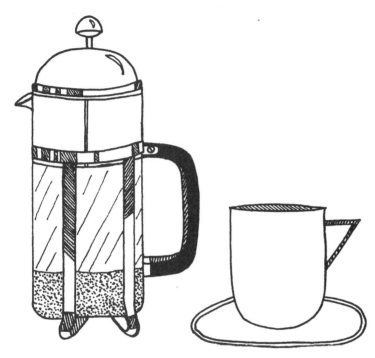

278 MAKE IT MILKY

Drinking a glass of milk could help reduce the severity of an asthma attack because the smoothness helps re-regulate breathing patterns. Adding turmeric, ginger or garlic to your milk is also thought to help reduce asthma.

279 BREATHE IN EUCALYPTUS

Eucalyptus essential oil is well known for helping to open up the airways, which is why it's such a good anti-asthma choice, especially for those whose asthma gets worse at night. Put a few drops on a paper towel or cloth and leave on a pillow or beside your bed while you sleep, or add to your bath or a steam inhalation.

280 MAKE YOUR OWN MEDICINE

To 2 cups water add 1 stick of cinnamon, 2 tablespoons chopped fresh thyme, the juice of 1 lime, 3 heads of garlic, peeled, and 1 small red onion. Place all the ingredients in a saucepan and bring to the boil, then add another cup of cold water and simmer until the mixture has reduced by half. Cool, strain and drink ½ to 1 cup, warm or cooled and sweetened with honey, three times a day.

277 GRAB A COFFEE

If you don't have your inhaler, a strong black coffee (as strong as you can take it) is a good way to help lessen an asthma attack because the caffeine helps open the blood vessels in the airways, reducing breathlessness. Make sure you don't add milk or cream, though, which could reduce the effectiveness.

281 RADISH REMEDY

Blitz ½ cup honey, ¼ cup lemon juice and 1 tablespoon chopped radish in a blender. Transfer to a saucepan and heat gently for 5 to 10 minutes. Seal and store in the fridge for three to five days. Take a spoonful daily.

282 GO FOR GINKGO

Ginkgo biloba is a herb that is widely believed to lessen the effects of asthma because it contains a compound called ginkgolide B, which helps increase bloodflow and prevents the airways from constricting. Ginkgo leaf extract can be taken as a tea or supplement, and the plant can be grown on a windowsill.

283 DRINK AN E TEA

Place 2 teaspoons each powdered Indian root (wild sarsaparilla), echinacea root and elecampane root in 2 cups hot water. Let the ingredients steep for 2 hours, then strain and store in an airtight container in the fridge. Drink a cup each morning and evening.

284 FIND THE FENUGREEK

Soak 1 teaspoon whole fenugreek seeds overnight. In the morning mix with 1 teaspoon fresh ginger juice in ½ cup hot water. Add honey to taste. Drink every morning to help combat asthma.

285 GET FLOWER POWER

A flower tea could help lessen asthma, particularly if it is allergic in origin. Mix 1 tablespoon each dried camomile flowers, echinacea root, mullein leaves and passionflower leaves in 500 ml (1 pint) hot water. Allow to steep for 5 minutes, then strain and drink as a tea to ease breathing.

286 JUICE WITH VITAMIN C

Mix 2 parts fresh carrot juice with 1 part fresh spinach juice and drink at the onset of an asthma attack to lessen symptoms. It is thought that the high levels of vitamin C in the vegetables help dilate the airways, making breathing easier.

287 GET HOLY

If you feel breathless holy basil (tulsi) can help to calm anxiety, which can contribute to breathing problems. Mix a few chopped leaves with honey and eat, or chew up the leaves mixed with rock salt or ground black pepper.

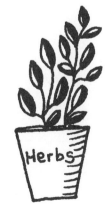

288 DECONGEST WITH ONION JUICE

Onion is good for getting rid of congestion on the chest. Juice 1 whole large onion with 1 teaspoon honey and a few grinds of fresh black pepper. Drink at the onset of symptoms to help alleviate breathing difficulties.

289 GET STEAMY

If you are suffering shortness of breath or an asthma attack, using steam might help open up your airways and make breathing easier. Including eucalyptus or lavender essential oils could speed up the process. Lean over a bowl of hot water to inhale the steam, or shut yourself in the bathroom with the shower on hot.

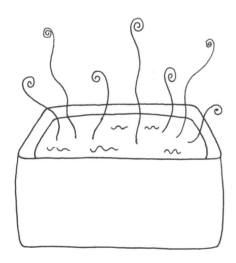

EMPHYSEMA

290 CHEW THE CURE

Chewing 2 to 3 cloves fresh garlic every day has been shown to be effective in treating emphysema naturally because of the powerful anti-inflammatory effects. Do this before every meal, if possible, or juice fresh garlic and add to other fruit or vegetable juices.

291 TAKE A TEASPOON OF JUICE

Drink 1 teaspoon of lemon or lime juice five times a day, spaced equally throughout, to help reduce the effects of emphysema. The acidity and high vitamin levels of the juice are thought to help lessen symptoms.

292 CHOOSE AN ANISEED CUBE

Aniseed has expectorant properties and is a folk cure for emphysema. Add 8 to 10 drops of aniseed oil to a sugar cube (brown sugar, if possible) and eat daily to help reduce emphysema.

293 ACT WITH AMARANTH

Amaranth is a green leafy vegetable with high levels of vitamins C and E, thought to help fight emphysema. Juice a handful of fresh amaranth leaves and add honey to taste. Take daily, preferably in the morning.

BRONCHITIS & COPD

294 ALMOND AND CITRUS INFUSION

Grind almonds in a pestle and mortar to make 1 tablespoon almond powder. Mix with 1 cup lemon or orange juice, then take the infusion once every evening to help reduce the pain and discomfort of bronchitis.

295 PEPPER AND GINGER MEDICINE

Mix equal amounts of ground black pepper, ginger and dried red pepper in a jar and store, covered, in a cool dark place. Add ½ teaspoon of the mixture to 1 cup of warm water, and drink three times a day.

296 LICK YOUR LIQUORICE

Put ½ teaspoon of liquorice root in a cup of boiling water and steep for 10 minutes, then strain and drink. Drink three times a day for a week.

297 MIX A MUSTARD PASTE

Mix up a paste of equal amounts of mustard powder, flour and water, and spread over the chest area. Make sure you do a patch test first to check for reactions. Leave on for 30 minutes, then rinse away.

298 GET FRANK ABOUT COUGHING

If you have a hacking cough, carry around a hand-kerchief with a few drops of frankincense essential oil – if your cough hurts or hacks, simply inhale the fumes.

299 TAKE REGULAR TEA

Tea can give COPD (Chronic Obstructive Pulmonary Disease) sufferers relief from tightening in the chest because it contains high levels of theophylline, which is the basic building block of many medical remedies. Take 3 to 4 cups a day to help breathing.

300 CHEW COMFREY

Chewing on comfrey leaves is a good choice for COPD because it stimulates the growth of new cells, inhibits the cough reflex and soothes inflammation in damaged lung tissues. Check with your doctor before eating, then try to include raw leaves in your diet daily.

301 SPIN FOR SPINACH

Blend a handful of fresh spinach leaves, 500 ml (1 pint) water and 1 teaspoon honey in a food processor. Drink every day to help cure bronchitis.

FOOD INTOLERANCES

302 EAT COCOA

Don't panic if you're lactose intolerant. Studies have shown that cocoa powder and sugar may help the body digest lactose more efficiently by slowing down the rate at which the stomach empties, thus reducing the lactose load on the body at one time. At last, a valid reason for eating chocolate! Chocolate milk is a good choice too.

303 SUCK A SARDINE

Sardines are high in calcium, which you may lack if you're not eating dairy products because of your lactose intolerance. Eat them regularly, along with salmon, broccoli, kale and spinach.

304 FIGHT IT WITH FLAX

Gluten sensitivity may cause some level of inflammation of the intestinal wall, which can lead to pain, bloating and discomfort. Ingesting 2 teaspoons flaxseeds at least once a day could help, as the seeds are completely gluten-free and rich in omega-3 fatty acids – a key force against inflammation.

305 YOKE UP A YOGURT

Because of the specific enzymes and cultures it contains, live (active culture) yogurt – although naturally high in lactose – is much easier to digest because part of the lactose has already started to break down. Try to include it in your diet.

306 PICK PEPPERMINT

Peppermint tea is known to help solve digestive problems because it contains high levels of menthol. To make tea, add 1 to 2 teaspoons dried peppermint leaves to a cup, pour in boiling water, and steep for 5 minutes. Strain, then drink to reduce symptoms.

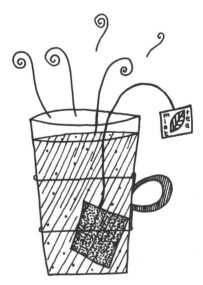

HICCUPS

307 MAKE IT MAGNESIUM

If your hiccups won't go with breath holding or any other simple cure, it might help to take an antacid, but make sure you choose one containing magnesium, which is known to decrease irritation.

308 HIT THE HONEY

Next time you have hiccups, try swallowing a teaspoon of honey. This is thought to work by filling the mouth with a sweet flavour, which helps the body stop hiccupping to 'concentrate' on the new item.

309 GET SOUR

In the same way that sugar or honey might help reduce hiccups – by filling the mouth with flavour – so might very sour tastes. Try sucking on a lemon or lime, or drinking a cold glass of pineapple or grapefruit juice.

310 GO GINGERLY

Sucking on a small piece of ginger is thought to be a good hiccup remedy – try crystallized ginger or root ginger, if your mouth can bear the strong taste. Alternatively, drink a ginger infusion.

311 SWALLOW SOME SEEDS

Simply swallowing a teaspoon full of dill seeds is thought to help get rid of hiccups. The seeds are an interesting texture for your mouth to deal with and that combined with the strong taste of the dill can shock the body into stopping.

312 MAKE MINE A MUSTARD

A good cure for hiccups is to put some mustard on your finger or a spoon, then place it on the back of your tongue and swallow it. The shock to your digestive system should help the hiccups disappear for good. You can also use cayenne pepper or chilli sauce.

313 DRINK SOME VINEGAR

Next time you have hiccups, try drinking vinegar (either straight white vinegar or from a jar of onions or pickles). The vinegar is thought to help reduce cramping, helping to dispel the irritating hiccup.

314 BE SWEET

Sugar is thought to be a good hiccup cure – try sucking a teaspoon of sugar with a few drops of water added to it, or if that is too sweet for you, add some to a slice of lemon or lime and suck. Aim for the back of the tongue, where sour tastes are detected.

315 SCARE YOUR SYSTEM WITH NUTS

Eating a teaspoon of peanut butter might not seem like the obvious hiccup cure, but many people believe the combination of salt and sweet helps 'confuse' the body into not thinking about hiccups. If you don't like peanut butter, try a tablespoon of yogurt with a pinch of salt.

316 ICE IT AWAY

Drink a glass of cold water, preferably with ice in it, as cold as you can bear. The cold is thought to 'shock' the body into stopping hiccups. Alternatively, you could apply an ice pack to the back of the neck, which will force a deep breath that may stop the hiccups.

DIARRHOEA

317 RICE TO THE OCCASION

Boil ¼ cup of brown rice in water for at least 30 minutes, preferably 45 minutes, then eat the rice and drink the water. The high levels of vitamin B are thought to give relief from diarrhoea.

318 SIP GINGER

Ease abdominal pain and stop your intestines cramping by drinking ginger tea. Alternate ginger tea with peppermint tea throughout the day to help reduce symptoms and help your intestines recover.

319 SIP BROTH

Thin chicken broth is a great way to replace lost body fluids and provide energy without causing the gut to become more inflamed or sore. Take small amounts regularly and try to drink it warm rather than hot. Homemade is best, with some salt.

ACID REFLUX OR HEARTBURN

320 GULP IT DOWN

At the very first sign of acid reflux appearing, take a full glass of water and drink it straight down – it's important not to sip, but gulp it down as fast as possible, which can help flush through the painful juices.

321 SUCK IT AWAY

Anything that increases the flow of saliva down through your digestive system is thought to help prevent reflux – chew on gum, a sweet or a piece of mint or ginger to help stimulate saliva flow and reduce pain.

322 EAT AN APPLE

Apples contain high levels of pectin, which is thought to bind up excess stomach acid, thus stopping reflux. Eat a slice of apple at times you are prone to heartburn or at the first flicker of pain, or drink apple juice if you don't like the crunch.

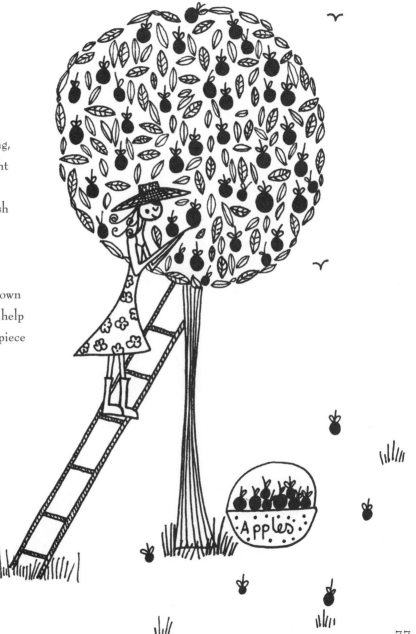

324 FUNNEL YOUR FENNEL

Fennel tea is a great choice for heartburn because it helps soothe and calm the digestive tract. Make fennel tea by steeping ½ to 1 teaspoon of fennel seeds in boiling water for 5 to 10 minutes. Strain and drink. Add a few drops of peppermint oil for added benefits.

325 TAKE SOME TEA

Camomile tea is a good way to help reduce the pain of heartburn and acid reflux for two reasons – one, it helps muscles relax and two, it has high levels of calcium, which can help settle the stomach.

326 JUICE IT UP

Raw vegetable juices are useful anti-reflux remedies because they help tame acid in the stomach. Choose carrot, beetroot or celery juice and add a pinch of fresh marjoram, basil or ginger to enhance the healing effects.

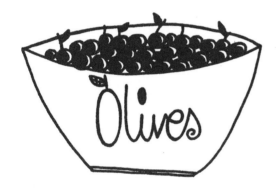

323 EAT OLIVES

After a meal, instead of reaching for the chocolate, have a couple of green or black olives in olive oil instead. The olives are naturally oily, which helps to coat the stomach and reduce pain. You can also eat them at the onset of pain, or take a teaspoon of olive oil instead.

327 A TEASPOON OF MUSTARD

Mustard might not seem the obvious choice for helping to reduce the pain of acid reflux, but taking a teaspoon of mustard can help pain disappear straight away. If you don't like the taste, mix it with some water and drink as a shot, or use ginger tea instead.

INDIGESTION

328 PICK UP A PINEAPPLE

Pineapple contains enzymes which can help you digest your food more easily – finish every meal with 125 ml (4 fl oz) fresh pineapple juice to help prevent indigestion developing later in the day.

329 BAKE IT AWAY

Mix up equal parts of bicarbonate of soda (baking soda) and water and take a tablespoonful to help reduce the pain of indigestion.

330 CHEW RAW POTATO

Potato has been used as an instant remedy to help prevent indigestion – at the first sign of pain simply chew thoroughly and swallow a small piece of raw potato.

331 GET A GRAPE

Grapes and grapefruit are both thought to be able to help indigestion. For grapes, simply eat a handful, making sure you chew well, after meals. For grapefruit, peel the skin into small pieces (avoiding the white pith), dry and take a spoonful to relieve symptoms.

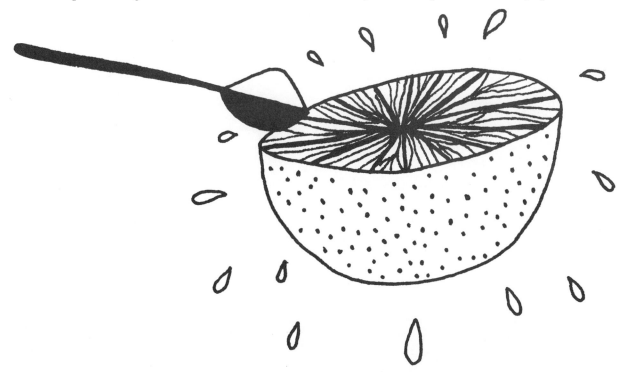

332 PICK SOME PARSLEY

There's a reason why parsley is often served as a garnish with meals – to help combat the signs of indigestion. Chew a sprig of parsley or take ¼ to ½ teaspoon of dried parsley and follow with a glass of water.

333 ASAFOETIDA FOR INDIGESTION

Mix up a homemade indigestion remedy. Add 1 teaspoon each of asafoetida, cumin seed powder and rock salt to 250 ml (8 fl oz) buttermilk, then add some crushed coriander (cilantro) leaves. Leave for 10 minutes, then drink. Repeat twice a day.

334 MAKE MINE MELON

Freshly juiced cantaloupe or honeydew makes a delicious, slushy drink that will clear the intestines and liven up the whole digestive tract. It is also excellent for weight loss and to relieve bloating.

335 CHEW CELERY

Celery is a well known indigestion cure because it is an 'alkaline' food, which relieves acid build-up in the stomach. Simply chomp on a celery stick, making sure you chew thoroughly, at the onset of indigestion pain.

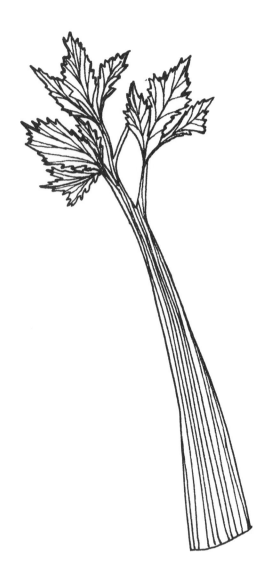

NAUSEA

336 ICE YOUR HEAD

Holding an ice pack to your forehead can help reduce nausea by affecting the nerves underlying the skin of the face, which can help reduce symptoms of nausea. Sit still for several minutes and repeat whenever necessary.

337 CHEW YOUR HERBS

The best things to chew to help prevent nausea are fresh mint, parsley, lemon or ginger root. You could also make a strong tea from these if you prefer.

338 MISO GREAT!

Miso soup is a great cure for nausea as the salt helps prevent that sick feeling. If you prefer, you can add some raw ginger to the soup to add flavour and boost the antinausea effects.

339 WHAT A GRIND

Grind up cumin seeds to make ½ teaspoon and take to prevent nausea. Follow with a glass of water and repeat once or twice a day to minimize symptoms. You can also mash or juice 3 slices cucumber, add sugar and water to taste, and drink.

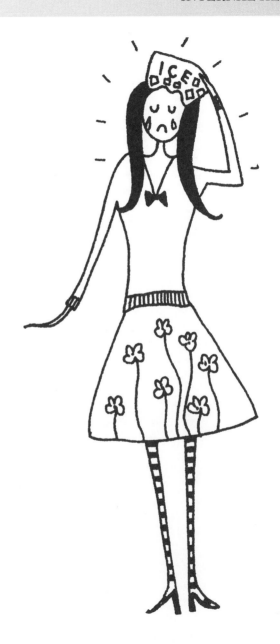

340 CRACK UP

Dry crackers or oatcakes are good for beating nausea as they taste bland and help mop up excess saliva and stomach acids which may be causing the symptoms. Try eating ¼ to ½ a cracker at the onset of nausea, eating more if necessary.

341 GET A BERRY CURE

Eating a bowl of fresh raspberries first thing in the morning on an empty stomach can help reduce nausea. If you don't like fresh raspberries you can try drinking raspberry or raspberry leaf tea (but beware of this if you're pregnant).

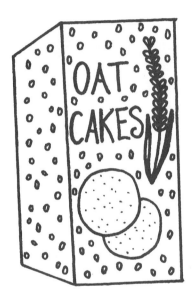

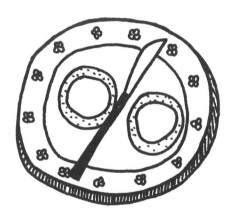

CONSTIPATION

342 SAY IT WITH SENNA

Senna is a common garden plant with natural laxative properties. Simply eat the raw senna seeds from inside the pod (about 1 teaspoonful) if you need to get things moving.

343 BE A PRUNE

Prune juice and stewed prunes are a good constipation cure – simply eat them twice a day if you want to loosen up your bowel movements.

344 EAT EPSOM

Epsom salts can be poisonous if taken in large quantities but in low dilutions they can act as a laxative. Simply add ¼ teaspoon Epsom salts to 125 ml (4 fl oz) water, mix well and drink.

345 OLIVE OIL AND ORANGE DRINK

Mix ¼ cup olive oil with ¼ cup freshly squeezed orange juice, and drink to relieve the symptoms of constipation. Make sure you drink a glass of water about 30 minutes later to ensure rehydration.

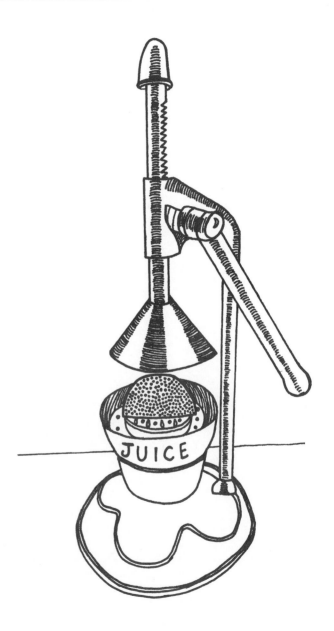

346 CONCOCTION FOR CONSTIPATION

If you want to help relieve the signs of constipation, combine equal amounts of freshly juiced carrot juice, apple juice and mango juice, then add a dash of prune juice. Drink a glass a day to help loosen bowels.

347 FIX IT WITH FIGS

Soak 2 fresh figs in water overnight, then in the morning eat the figs with natural live (active culture) yogurt and drink the water they have soaked in (add a little warm water to make it more palatable if you prefer.

348 AN APPLE A DAY

Apples are thought to be mild laxatives and they are a great choice to consume daily to help permanently loosen bowels to a comfortable level. Choose lower-sugar varieties such as Cox and Russett for best effects.

349 EAT BROWN RICE

A high-fibre alternative to white rice, the fibres present in brown rice increase bowl movement, thus helping to reduce constipation.

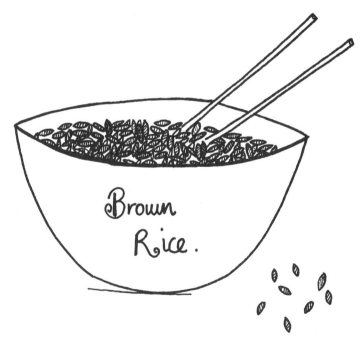

HAEMORRHOIDS

350 WHITE RADISH JUICE

Also known as daikon or mooli, the white radish is thought to be a good cure for haemorrhoids and is much milder than the small red variety. Drink a radish juice sweetened with a little honey every morning and evening (prepare in a juicer or blender, or chop and squeeze manually). For a topical preparation, grate white radish and add enough milk to form a paste, then smooth over the affected area.

351 CHOOSE CORIANDER (CILANTRO)

Coriander (cilantro) is a good choice for relief from piles. Go for a double whammy by drinking coriander juice and using coriander paste as a balm. To make the paste mix 1 teaspoon powdered dried mango seeds into 1 tablespoon coriander juice and apply to the affected area.

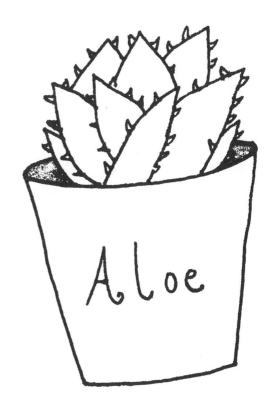

352 KNOW YOUR ONIONS

Soak an onion in warm, sweetened water overnight and eat it the next day to help relieve piles from the inside out. Warm it gently on the stove or in a microwave and add a little more sugar or honey to make it more palatable, if you prefer.

353 SALVE-ATION FOR PILES

Make a topical cream or ointment to help provide relief from piles. Neat aloe vera gel or witch hazel are good choices, or create a salve with echinacea root, myrrh or white oak. Alternatively, mix the powdered ingredient with olive oil to form an ointment.

INCONTINENCE

354 CRUSH A CRANBERRY

Cranberry juice is well known for aiding urinary problems, including bladder infections which might lie at the root of incontinence. Drink a glass every day to help flush through the system and reduce infection.

355 SWAP YOUR DRINKS

Instead of drinking tea and coffee, the caffeine in which could actually make your incontinence worse, swap your morning drinks for a glass of juice instead – choose grape, cranberry, cherry and apple, which help soothe the bladder lining, rather than citrus juices.

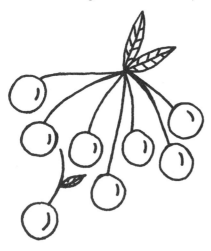

IRRITABLE BOWEL SYNDROME

356 BRING ON THE BRAN

Increasing fibre levels is beneficial for almost all gastrointestinal complaints and oat bran is a very good choice because it is bland, which means it can also soothe the intestinal lining. Eat oatmeal every day in as mild a form as possible and expect to see results in a month. Make sure you drink water too, especially if you are increasing fibre intake.

357 CHOOSE CABBAGE

Cabbage contains enzymes and compounds which soothe the intestine – wash the leaves of a cabbage in boiling water to warm them up a little, then put through a juicer or blender. Or cook the cabbage in a small amount of water until mushy and then mash and eat.

358 GO DARK

Lettuce is a great choice for IBS sufferers as it helps relieve the symptoms of bloating and gas; choose the darkest varieties possible, which will have a more powerful effect.

359 REDUCE PAIN WITH FENNEL

Fennel seeds can help reduce pain by limiting intestinal spasms and reducing fat in the system, thus helping to reduce mucus production. Make a tea by steeping 1 teaspoon of fennel seeds in 1 cup boiling water for 5 to 10 minutes, then strain and drink. Alternatively add fennel seeds to vegetable juices such as carrot, cabbage and pear or sprinkle them over salads and in soups.

360 PICK PEPPERMINT

Many studies have found peppermint to be useful in combating the symptoms of IBS, particularly when peppermint oil is used because it helps stop cramping and diarrhoea. Make a tea using 1 to 2 teaspoons of dried peppermint in a cup of boiling water, steep for 10 minutes, and then drink.

361 A BAKING DRINK

If you have trapped wind or gas problems, add 1 teaspoon baking powder to a glass of water and drink immediately. It will relieve the pain by helping the gas to dissipate rather than building up in specific areas.

362 WATER IT DOWN

Next time you begin to suffer wind pains, drink a cup of water, as hot as you can stand it, mixed with the juice from half a lemon. This will help free up trapped wind and ease pain and cramping.

363 DRINK BASIL LEAF TEA

Basil leaf tea is good for reducing gas – simply crush and roll some leaves in your hand, add to a teapot, pour over boiling water and steep for 10 to 15 minutes. Drink a cup two to three times a day for gas relief.

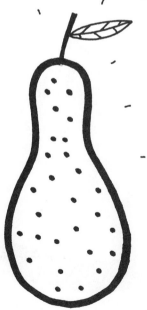

364 JUICE YOUR CARROTS AND PEARS

Carrots are a great choice for helping with IBS and the best way to eat them is freshly juiced. As they're not juicy themselves, add some sweet pear juice to make the taste and texture better and boost the healing effects, or simply eat them lightly steamed or boiled, if you prefer.

HIGH BLOOD PRESSURE

365 WATERMELON JUICE

The juice of the seeds of watermelon contains an ingredient that is thought to dilate the capillaries. It acts on the kidneys and thereby lowers the blood pressure. Grind watermelon seeds and soak them in a cup of boiling water for an hour. Then stir, strain and drink. Take four doses daily. Watermelon juice is also beneficial.

366 ADD CONDIMENTS TO YOUR FOOD

Parsley, cayenne pepper and coriander (cilantro) are all useful in combating high blood pressure. Use them liberally in your cooking, preferably in as raw a form as possible to maximize benefits.

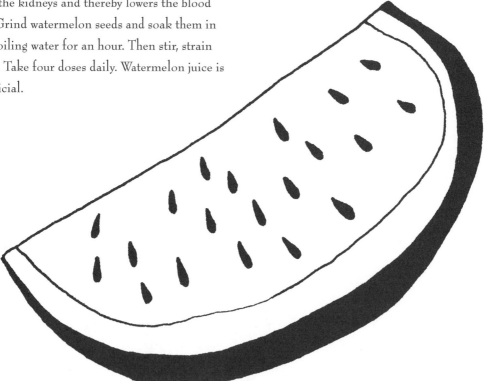

367 LOVE YOUR LEMONS

For a great home remedy to lower blood pressure, drink the juice of ½ lemon every day mixed with warm water. This is a great substitute for coffee as it's an energy booster as well.

368 VINEGAR YOUR SYSTEM

That old favourite, vinegar, is back and this time it's to help you lower blood pressure. Mix 2 to 3 tablespoons of cider vinegar with warm water and drink daily to help lower blood pressure naturally.

369 DON'T MISS THE MISTLETOE

Instead of throwing away your mistletoe after Christmas this year, dry the leaves and store them in an airtight container. Use 1 teaspoon dried mistletoe leaves to make a tea to help lower blood pressure.

370 GET HERBAL

Make your own blood pressure lowering herbal tea using hawthorn berries (you can also use hawthorn extract, if you prefer, and take directly). Mix 1 teaspoon crushed dried hawthorn berries with 2 teaspoons dried yarrow in the juice of ½ lime. Add 1 cup of boiling water, steep for 15 minutes, then strain and drink. Take two or three times a day.

HIGH CHOLESTEROL

371 DRINK GARLIC JUICE

Garlic is a great way to lower cholesterol naturally because of all the natural enzymes it contains. Extract the juice of 2 cloves by crushing in a pestle and mortar and drink a spoonful every day. Not only does garlic lower cholesterol, it also affects the balance of 'good' and 'bad' cholesterol, making you healthier.

372 SNACK ON ALMONDS

Snacking on a handful of almonds once a day could help you to reduce cholesterol levels naturally as the nuts contain substances which help strip out cholesterol from the bloodstream. Studies also suggest that eating walnuts four times a week could have similar effects.

373 HAVE SOME HONEY

Honey has long been believed to help lower cholesterol if taken as 1 teaspoon a day, either plain or mixed with warm water, along with 1 teaspoon of fresh lime or lemon juice or cider vinegar.

374 GET YOUR OATS

Simply the most powerful remedy for cholesterol is to eat oats every day – make them with water rather than milk and eat at least half a cup every morning, which has been shown to lower cholesterol by up to 9%.

375 STICK TO SOYABEANS

Eating soyabeans several times a week could help you fight off cholesterol build-up by altering the levels of LDL and HDL stored in the body's systems. Aim to eat them two or three times a week for best effects.

376 TURMERIC AND AUBERGINE DIP RECIPE

Turmeric is thought to have cholesterol-lowering effects – get twice the dose by mixing 1 teaspoon turmeric with 1 cooked mashed aubergine (eggplant) and use as a dip or spread.

377 RHUBARBS AND YOGURT

Make a cholesterol-busting rhubarb fool using stewed rhubarb, mashed and mixed with the same amount of low-fat natural live (active culture) yogurt, then chilled in the fridge. Rhubarb lowers cholesterol and yogurt helps balance the blood system.

378 ASK FOR ARTICHOKE

Eating artichoke is not only healthy, it can actually lower cholesterol levels all on its own. Eat lightly cooked on its own or blitzed into soups for best effects.

379 PLACE THE PECTIN

Foods containing high levels of pectin such as carrots and apples are a great way to lower cholesterol as they help bind up damaging levels of cholesterol in the bloodstream and alter the balance of 'good' and 'bad' cholesterol.

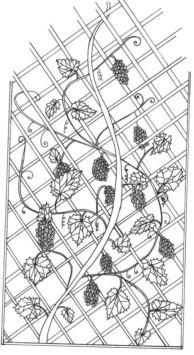

380 GET A GRAPE

Red grapes have high levels of antioxidants, which are thought to help lower cholesterol naturally. Eat them raw or juice them (with skins) for a liquid treat. Shop-bought red grape juice will work too, but might not be as potent without the skins.

POOR CIRCULATION

381 EAT YOUR ONIONS

Eating onions every day can help to improve the circulation as well as relax muscles, reducing stress. Onions are actually easier to digest if they are partially cooked, so grilling or roasting lightly works well.

382 BOOST YOUR WARMTH

Drinking up a warming tea can help boost blood circulation to your extremities (as opposed to caffeinated drinks, which can actually reduce circulation). Infuse fresh ginger and cayenne pepper into hot water and drink to boost blood flow.

383 GO FOR GINSENG

Ginseng is a great supplement to take if you suffer from circulation problems – not only does it work to regulate sugar levels to help with diabetes, it also reduces cholesterol and has anticlotting properties.

384 HAVE A TIPPLE

Red wine is known for its ability to enable the circulatory system to function optimally. Infuse a bottle of wine with rosemary flowers for a more potent effect, then take 60 ml (2 fl oz) daily or every other day.

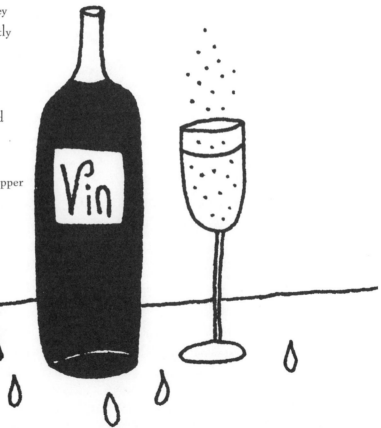

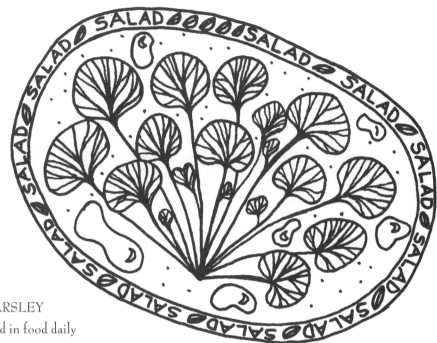

DIABETES

385 WATERCRESS AND PARSLEY

Parsley is a natural diabetic and used in food daily can help to lower blood-sugar levels. Watercress contains similar levels of insulin-levelling chemicals, so is a great choice for salads and soups.

386 BATHE IN SALT

Taking a warm salt bath won't help your diabetes get better, but it can help reduce the itching of one of the major side effects – dry, flaky skin. Add a couple of handfuls of salt to a warm bath and soak for 20 minutes. Use extra salt as an exfoliant to boost circulation as well.

387 CINNAMON SPICE

Cinnamon is high in magnesium, which is essential for many of the body's key systems, including insulin production. For Type Two diabetes, adding ½ teaspoon ground cinnamon a day to your diet could have beneficial results. Sprinkle it on buttered toast, apple slices, oatmeal or in yogurt. Alternatively add a cinnamon stick to ordinary tea to make a chai tea.

388 RE-SUGAR WITH PEANUTS

If you're feeling like your blood sugar may be low, a great way to help your system plump up sugar levels naturally is to eat a couple of crackers covered in peanut butter for a low sugar, protein-carbohydrate snack. Avoid brands that contain added sugar or glucose.

389 FRESHEN UP WITH FENUGREEK

Fenugreek is thought to help diabetes by lengthening the amount of time that the body takes to digest sugars, thus regulating blood sugar. Take the seeds consistently with meals as a tea or supplement.

390 BE SAGE

Sage is a great choice for diabetes as it is thought to boost the production of insulin in the body as well as increase liver function, which in turn can help regulate sugar levels. Use the fresh leaves to make tea and drink once a day on an empty stomach.

391 BE A VIRGIN LOVER

Studies have shown that extra-virgin olive oil could have a beneficial effect on blood sugar levels, helping to reduce them. Use an oil mister and make sure you don't use too much as this can cause you to gain weight, which is a risk factor for diabetes.

LIVER PROBLEMS

392 GET PRICKLY

Milk thistle is one of the best-known herbal treatments for helping your liver to detoxify and cleanse naturally. Take daily as directed and supplement with dandelion for a stronger remedy.

393 BREW UP BILBERRY

Bilberries are thought to help lower blood sugar and regulate insulin levels. To make the tea, place 1 tablespoon dried bilberry leaves in 1 cup of boiling water, steep for 10 minutes, then strain and drink. Take three times a day for best effects.

394 OPT FOR OREGANO

Oregano tea is a good choice for liver function because it contains antioxidants and acts as a detoxifier. Infuse dried oregano with lemon leaves and steep for 5 to 10 minutes. Strain and drink.

395 FIX IT WITH FIG

Wash 3 to 4 leaves of the sacred fig (*Ficus religiosa*), sprinkle over sugar, mash thoroughly and mix with ½ cup water. Drink twice daily. If you can't find sacred fig, you can substitute white radish leaves.

396 LIME AND PAPAYA SEED MEDICINE

Take the black papaya seeds from the inside of fresh papaya and grind in a pestle and mortar or a liquidizer to get 1 tablespoon juice. Combine with 1 teaspoon fresh lime juice and take once daily for a month to help cleanse your liver.

397 GET HOT TO TROT

Hot mustard powder is a great liver cleanser, especially if you suffer jaundice. Use mustard powder or powder your own by grinding yellow mustard seeds, then smear on a banana (which contains high levels of potassium) and eat once a day.

398 COOK WITH KARELA

Also known by the names bitter gourd and bitter melon, karela (*Momordica charantia*) is available from Asian food stores and is a traditional Ayurvedic cure for liver problems. Simply juice the fruit and drink ½ cup on an empty stomach. Alternatively, boil in small amounts of water for at least 30 minutes, then strain and drink the water (it should taste bitter).

399 FISH FOR FRUCTOSE

Fructose sugars are thought to help give the body energy while being much easier for the liver to cope with than complex sugars. Choose fresh fruit and vegetables wherever possible to give your liver a break. Home-grown varieties are the best but if you don't have the time or inclination to grow your own, buy organic from local farms.

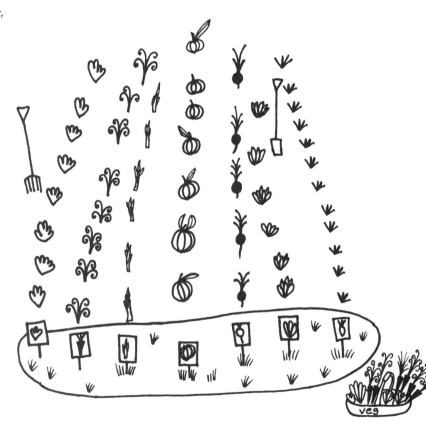

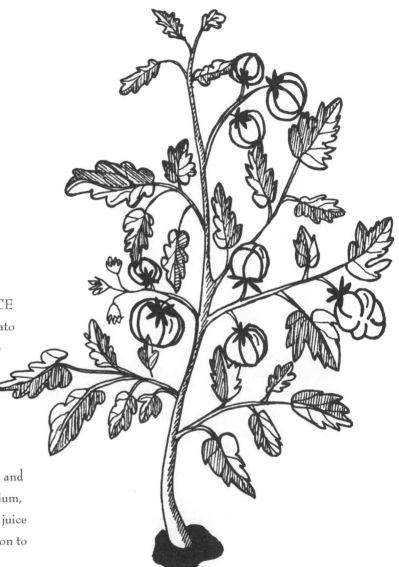

JAUNDICE

400 TOMATO JUICE FOR JAUNDICE

Drink 250 ml (8 fl oz) freshly squeezed tomato juice with a small pinch of salt to help reduce jaundice. Alternatively, add ½ teaspoon ginger juice and 1 teaspoon fresh lime juice to mint tea.

401 MASH YOUR BANANAS

Mash 1 ripe banana with 1 tablespoon honey and eat twice a day. This has high levels of potassium, which helps to boost liver function. Beetroot juice also serves the same purpose, mixed with lemon to improve the taste.

VARICOSE VEINS

402 JUICE VEINS AWAY

Drinking a combination of freshly squeezed carrot and spinach juice every day is thought to help varicose veins to heal because it contains high levels of vitamin E. Mix twice the amount of carrot juice to spinach, and drink a glass daily.

403 GO ON A WITCH HUNT

Witch hazel is a great choice if your varicose veins need attention as it's a natural astringent and also contains tannins and gallic acids to reduce pain and swelling. You can drink it as tea, but it's most potent when used as a compress.

404 BATHE IT AWAY

A bath containing a cupful of Epsom salts can ease varicose veins and encourage healing, especially if using as alternate warm and cool baths.

405 MASSAGE WITH LAVENDER

Using pure lavender essential oil, massage the veins in an upward direction towards the heart After a few minutes you'll begin to feel relief as the calming, healing effects of the lavender kick in.

406 ASK ST JOHN

St John's wort is a good healing cure for varicose veins – use olive oil infused with St John's wort flowers to massage over affected areas. To make, add a handful of the flowers to a small bottle of oil and leave, sealed, for two to three weeks out of sunlight. Alternatively drink an infusion of the flowers.

407 CALENDULA BODY BUTTER

Make your own tightening body butter using calendula. Mix together 2 cups fresh calendula flowers with a thick substrate like lard, butter or even your own moisturizing cream. Gently apply to the veins and leave to soak in.

408 RECKON ON ROSEMARY

Rosemary has similar healing effects to lavender, but the oil cannot be used alone so be sure to mix it with a carrier oil to avoid skin problems. Massage into affected veins (always upwards towards the heart) or drink as a tea.

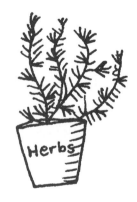

ANGINA

409 LOVE LEMONS

Lemon is thought to prevent the clogging of blood vessels by cholesterol, which may help in preventing angina. Try to take lemon every day in your diet – a good way is to use the fresh juice squeezed into hot or cold water, or on salads as a dressing.

410 BASE IT WITH BASIL

Basil leaves can reduce blood cholesterol levels and help protect the heart from continued damage. Mix 1 teaspoon of fresh basil juice with 1 teaspoon of honey and drink on an empty stomach.

411 GO FOR GARLIC

Garlic can help reduce cholesterol build-up in blood vessels, helping to prevent angina. Try to eat 2 cloves raw garlic every day, preferably on an empty stomach, to help fight against angina developing.

412 PICK PARSLEY

Parsley tea, taken two or three times a day, is a good natural remedy for angina. Let the fresh parsley steep for at least 10 minutes to get most beneficial effects, and drink warm.

413 HANG OUT FOR HAWTHORN

The dried fruits, flowers and leaves of the hawthorn plant have several uses. They can cause dilation of coronary vessels, which can promote blood flow and thus reduce pain from angina. Take as a liquid extract with meals, followed by a glass of water. Hawthorn berries can be eaten raw, but are quite tasteless.

414 OWN YOUR ONIONS

Onion juice is thought to help de-fuzz the arteries. Take 1 teaspoon of raw onion juice before you have breakfast every morning, then wait 30 minutes before eating or drinking anything else. A juicer is the best method to prepare, and 1 onion will yield 2 to 3 tablespoons of juice. The juice can be stored in the fridge for two to three days.

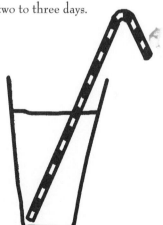

ARTHRITIS

415 PICK A POTATO

Potato juice is thought to help relieve the grinding pain of arthritis – extract the juice of a potato and fill a cup to halfway, then fill up the rest with warm water. Drink before breakfast on an empty stomach to help relieve pain.

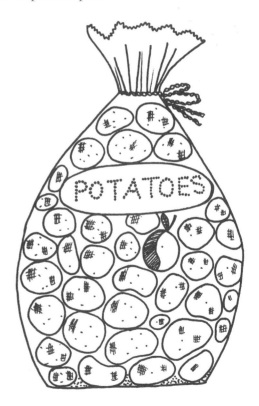

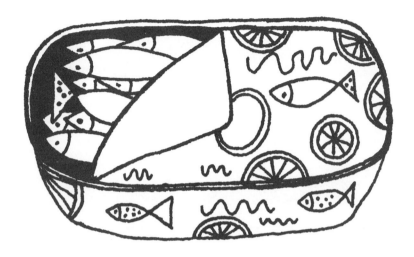

416 GET OUT THE OLIVE OIL

Warm olive oil is a great way to help reduce arthritis pain. Simply cover warm hands in warmed olive oil and massage the affected area gently, applying upward pressure to help reduce pain. Better still, add a few drops of lavender, rosemary or thyme oils to add scent and aid relaxation.

417 RUB AWAY PAIN WITH VINEGAR

Heat 1 cup of cider vinegar in a saucepan or in the microwave until it is as hot as you can bear without burning. Now use your hands (or have someone else do it for you if the area is hard to reach) to gently massage it into the affected area for at least 10 minutes.

418 EAT FISH FOR FISH OILS

Fish oils are thought to be of great help in relieving the symptoms of arthritis because they allow the joints to lubricate themselves and therefore reduce pain and swelling. Any fish is a good choice – aim for three to four portions weekly.

419 SOOTHE WITH A JUNIPER SALT BATH

A sea salt bath is thought to help ease pain in the same way that sea swimming does. Lace your bath with healing juniper essential oils to help stimulate blood flow around joints and reduce pain. Alternatively, try lavender, camomile, cypress or lemon.

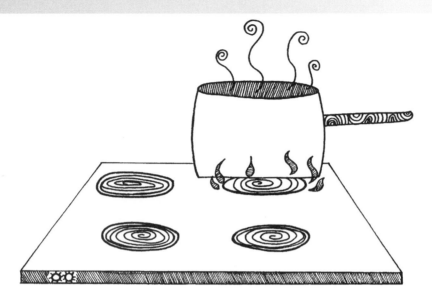

420 NOURISHING NETTLE SOUP

Make nettle soup using 1 chopped onion, 4 cloves chopped garlic, 3 cups fresh nettle tops, 1 tablespoon flour, 500 ml (1 pint) stock and 250 ml (½ pint) skimmed milk. Heat the onion and garlic in a little butter, stir in the flour then stock, stirring constantly. Add the nettle and cook for 10 to 15 minutes, until soft. Blend and stir in the milk. Drink a cup of the soup every day to help relieve the symptoms of arthritis.

421 GET THE FLAX

Flaxseed oil is a natural cure for arthritis. Add flaxseeds to your cereal, take flaxseed oil three times daily or grind up flaxseeds and sprinkle on any meal.

422 ASK FOR ALFALFA

Alfalfa has anti-inflammatory properties, so including it in your diet is a good choice if you suffer from arthritis pain. Make a tea by adding 1 teaspoon of alfalfa seeds to 1 cup of boiling water. Allow to steep for 10 minutes, then strain and drink.

423 CHECK WITH CINNAMON

Cinnamon is a powerful anti-inflammatory and using it in conjunction with honey makes it even more potent. Before breakfast every morning, add 1 teaspoon ground cinnamon to 1 tablespoon honey. mix and eat, either raw or combined with warm water as a drink.

424 ROOT OUT ARTHRITIS WITH GINGER

Ginger is thought to help protect against arthritis because it has powerful anti-inflammatory properties. Infuse the fresh root in hot water and drink as a tea first thing in the morning. Add lemon or honey to boost the anti-arthritis effects.

425 BLEND A CURE

Blend 1 cup honey with 10 cloves garlic and 1 cup apple cider vinegar. Transfer to a jar, cover and refrigerate for up to a week. Take 1 tablespoon a day, either raw or diluted in warm water.

426 LOOSEN JOINTS WITH COCONUT

There is some evidence that coconut oil can help reduce the pain of arthritis by helping to lubricate the joints. Ingest 1 teaspoon of coconut oil two to three times a day to lessen symptoms.

427 RAISIN A CURE

Soak golden raisins in just enough gin to cover them, cover and leave for 10 days in the fridge. Eat 6 to 10 raisins every day to help reduce arthritis pains.

428 WARM UP WITH MUSTARD OIL

Add 2 cloves garlic to a carrier base of hot mustard oil (available from supermarkets and Asian markets) – just enough to cover the garlic – and allow to infuse for several days. Then remove the garlic cloves and use the oil to massage areas affected by arthritis. The garlic-mustard oil will soothe pain, reduce inflammation and increase blood flow.

429 LAY ON A LEAF

For instant relief throughout the day peel off the outer layer of an aloe vera leaf, then heat up the inside gel in a microwave for 10 to 15 seconds. Apply the heated gel to the affected area, carefully wrap with a clean towel or gauze, and leave until it is completely cooled.

430 KEEP JOINTS COMFREY

Make up a cream containing 500 ml (1 pint) aqueous cream and 500 ml (1 pint) chopped comfrey leaves. Microwave for 8 to 10 minutes and then strain. Add 1 teaspoon each eucalyptus oil, camphor oil, arnica oil and vitamin E oil. Apply a teaspoon of the mixture to the affected area three times a day. Keep refrigerated between applications; it will last several months in the fridge.

431 SAY IT WITH CHERRIES

Cherries have powerful natural anti-inflammatory properties, which makes them a great choice for treating arthritis, particularly gout. Eat 225 g (½ lb) of cherries per day at the onset of problems for about a week and you should see great results.

432 PECK UP WITH PECTIN

To a glass of red or purple grape juice (make sure this is juice and not a flavoured drink), add 2 tablespoons fruit pectin (available from supermarkets). Mix together and drink once a day to help reduce arthritis pain.

433 USE ALOE

Mash and then strain enough juice from the aloe vera plant to make 1 teaspoon of aloe juice. Add this liquid to 250 ml (8 fl oz) orange juice or water and drink every morning before breakfast to help stave off arthritis pains.

434 ASH AND TEQUILA RUB

Chop or mash a rinsed Pick a handful of leaves from the common ash tree (*Fraxinus excelsior*). Rinse the leaves, then chop or mash them and mix with enough tequila to form a paste. Rub directly onto sore joints to help reduce pain and swelling.

RHEUMATISM

435 DRINK WITH CELERY SEED

Celery is a good choice for treating joint pain because it helps reduce inflammation. Crunching celery sticks is helpful, but consuming the extract of the seeds is more powerful. Available from health food stores, the liquid extract should be taken with plenty of juice or water at mealtimes. The recommended dosage is ½ teaspoon of the extract three times a day.

436 CREATE AN INVIGORATING CAMPHOR RUB

Make yourself a homemade massage rub for sore, painful joints. Add 4 drops each of eucalyptus oil and either menthol or peppermint oil to 1 tablespoon of camphor oil. Rub the ointment onto the affected joints at night before bed to help ease away pain.

437 ROAR FOR RHUBARB

Rhubarb has been shown to be good for rheumatism – simply pound raw rhubarb stems with a sprinkling of sugar and 1 tablespoon water. Take 1 teaspoon twice a day to help reduce pain and swelling.

438 CHOOSE BLACKCURRANT

Sprinkle a handful of fresh or dried blackcurrant leaves into a teapot and pour over boiling water. Allow to steep for 10 minutes and drink a cup twice a day. Marigold flowers, pansy flowers and dandelion can also be used.

439 COD LIVER AND ORANGE

Cod liver oil is thought to be helpful for all joint pain, including rheumatism. Mix 1 tablespoon into 250 ml (8 fl oz) orange juice, whisk and drink before bed for a pain-free night.

440 DIP INTO A BUCKET

Into a bucket or basin of warm water add salt or Epsom salts and several drops of rosemary essential oil. Soak the affected area in the solution for 10 to 15 minutes while relaxing to help ease pain.

441 GET LIMEY

Mix up 2 tablespoons of water with 1 tablespoon of freshly squeezed lime juice and drink every morning to help reduce rheumatic pain. You can substitute lemon juice if you prefer the taste, but lime is more powerful.

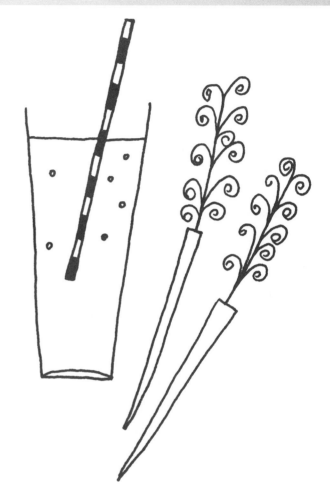

442 CARROT AND LEMON JUICE

Carrot juice and lemon juice, when used in combination, are thought to help reduce arthritis and rheumatism pain. Mix up the juices in equal amounts and take a tablespoonful every day.

MUSCLE SORENESS

443 PREVENT CRAMPING WITH CHICKEN BROTH

Drinking a cup of warm soup before heading out on a bike ride may not get you in the mood for exercise, but it's just the thing to help prevent muscle cramps later on. Consuming beef or chicken bouillon before you ride will help replace lost sodium and reduce cramping.

444 SOAK IT AWAY

Soaking in a bath of Epsom salts 24 hours after exercise can help reduce muscle cramps and soreness by providing magnesium that will assist in the healing of torn muscles. Add 2 cups of Epsom salts to a hot bath and soak away.

445 ROCK WITH ROSEMARY

Rosemary contains a mixture of anti-inflammatory substances and works through the skin to heal underlying tissues. Brew a pot of rosemary tea by pouring boiling water over a handful of fresh leaves. Allow to cool and use the strained liquid to soak a cloth. Apply the cloth compress to the affected area several times a day.

446 EAT A BANANA

As a potassium deficiency in tired muscles can lead to cramps, eating one or two bananas a day can help prevent post-exercise cramps.

447 DRINK MILK

Milk is a good choice if you want to cut down on cramps because it contains high levels of calcium, which can help muscles heal more quickly. Choose skimmed or semi-skimmed, in which the calcium is more readily available. Aim for two 250 ml (8 fl oz) glasses a day.

448 A PINE NEEDLE SOLUTION

Soak a bowl of pine needles overnight in just enough water to cover them. The next day, strain and use the water in your bath to relieve tired and sore muscles. Soak for 20 minutes, but avoid getting the water near your eyes as it might sting.

449 GET STONED

Remove the stone from a ripe avocado and grind it to a powder in a liquidizer or coffee grinder. Mix the resulting powder with enough surgical spirit (rubbing alcohol) to form a paste and use to rub on aches and pains to help them disappear.

450 TURN UP THE HEAT

Combine 2 cups sunflower or olive oil with 2 tablespoons habanero chilli powder and heat over a very low flame for around two hours, stirring occasionally. Strain through a muslin (cheesecloth) into a clean glass jar and use the oil to massage sore muscles. Mix in beeswax if you prefer a salve formulation.

451 MAKE IT MINTY

Combine a handful of fresh chopped mint with 2 to 3 tablespoons petroleum jelly (or even butter, if you prefer). Allow to infuse for several hours, then use the ointment on aching muscles to reduce pain and stiffness. Or try lard with camphor for a more pungent alternative.

452 USE AN ANCIENT CURE

An old Roman cure for muscle aches and pains is to have a hot mustard bath (sprinkle hot mustard powder into a hot bath), followed by a semi-hot lavender bath (using dried lavender flowers or 10 drops of lavender essential oil) and finally finishing with a cold shower. Soak for 15 minutes in each of the baths and shower briefly in the cold before drying.

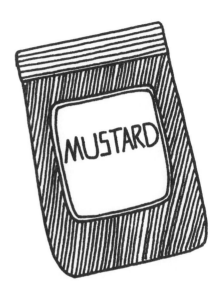

BACK & NECK PAIN

453 USE A MUSTARD POULTICE

If your pain is in the lower back area, mix up a healing poultice with dry white or yellow mustard powder and enough tequila to make a spreadable paste. Leave the mixture to warm up on a sunny windowsill for 30 minutes. Apply to the lower back, covering with a warm towel for 20 minutes before wiping off with paper towels.

454 PRESS YOUR ADVANTAGE

Add several drops of eucalyptus and lavender essential oils to a small saucepan of hot water. Soak a cloth or small towel in the water, wring out excess water, and apply as a compress to the sore area of your back or neck to reduce pain.

455 RELAX MUSCLES WITH CAMOMILE

Stress can make muscles feel knotted, which may exacerbate back pain. Camomile tea is not only a natural way to relax, it also has muscle relaxant qualities which help reduce pain. Steep 1 tablespoon fresh camomile flowers in 1 cup hot water for 15 minutes, then strain and drink two to three cups a day.

456 DRINK AWAY YOUR PAIN

Ginger isn't only good for curing nausea, it's also great for back pain as it's an anti-inflammatory. Drink ginger tea using the root of ginger (do not use ground ginger) three times a day for pain relief. Simply pour hot water over fresh chopped ginger root and leave to infuse before straining and drinking.

457 CHOOSE CAPSAICIN

Capsaicin cream is made from the same substance that makes chilli peppers hot and it also acts as a pain reliever when used as an ointment. Apply directly to the sore area for temporary relief.

458 SOCK IT TO PAIN

Fill a clean, thick sock with a cup of uncooked rice, tie a knot in the end and heat in the microwave for 30 to 60 seconds on a medium heat. Check the temperature and apply to the sore area of your back for 5 to 10 minutes. Try to remain still while the heat works to relieve pain.

459 BE A DEVIL

Devil's claw (available from herbal stores and some supermarkets) is a herb that originates in South Africa, where it has been used for centuries to help reduce bone and joint pain. Take as a tea or supplement at the onset of pain.

460 TAKE WHITE WILLOW

White willow bark (*Salix alba*) is the original source of aspirin, a commonly used painkiller. Use white willow to cope with and prevent conditions involving pain and inflammation, like osteoarthritis and back pain. Buy as an extract from herbal stores (and take according to the instructions on the package) or make your own remedy by soaking the bark in a bottle of oil (for a topical rub). Alternatively, dry and use a teaspoon in a cup of hot water to make a tea.

BURSITIS

461 MAKE A CAYENNE COMPRESS

Add 1 teaspoon cayenne pepper to 1 cup apple cider vinegar and simmer for 15 minutes. Allow to cool to hand-hot. Soak a cloth in the vinegar, wring out any excess, and hold on the affected area to reduce swelling.

462 RAISE YOUR RADISH

Horseradish can be used to make a topical poultice to apply directly to the site of pain. Grate enough for 2 tablespoons horseradish root and place in an old sock, stocking or laundry bag. Moisten the bag with water and apply directly to the affected area.

463 BE ARMED WITH ARNICA

Arnica is a great anti-inflammatory and you can use the ointment to rub directly onto the wounded area, or add a few drops of arnica oil into a carrier oil like sesame or olive and use to massage instead.

464 DRINK POTATO WATER

Before you go to bed, grate a potato and add it to a cup of water. Soak overnight in the fridge. In the morning, strain and drink the leftover water before breakfast. This is thought to prevent fluid build-up, reducing bursitis.

CARPAL TUNNEL SYNDROME

465 REDUCE SWELLING WITH MINT

Japanese mint oil (available from online stores) can help carpal tunnel syndrome by reducing swelling. Apply a few drops to the wrist in the morning and cover with a warm wet compress for 5 minutes. Repeat in the evening but using a cold wet compress.

466 HAVE A LAVENDER SOAK

For numbness, tingling and pain in the hand and wrist, add a few drops of lavender essential oil to warm water and soak your hand for 30 minutes.

OSTEOPOROSIS

467 PEANUTS FOR GOOD BONES

Magnesium is a vital component of bones and is required to strengthen and preserve them. Get a daily magnesium dose to help your bones by sprinkling peanuts on your salad or cereal for extra nutrients and crunch, snacking on a handful of raw peanuts, or dipping vegetable and fruit slices into peanut butter (choose unsweetened, if possible).

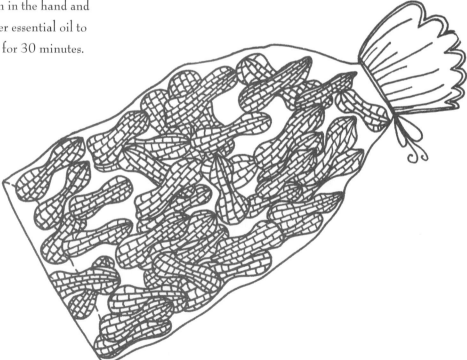

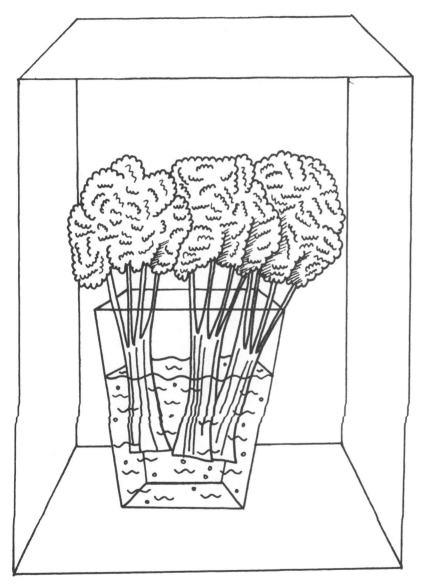

468 BAG SOME BROCCOLI

Eating just ½ cup of broccoli a day will help you get a huge dose of vitamins, including vitamin K, a lack of which has been linked to osteoporosis in post–menopausal women. Eat it steamed or microwaved for best results.

469 DIG IN TO DANDELION

Dandelion leaf tea is thought to help boost bone density, making it a great choice for osteoporosis. Drink 2 to 3 cups a day for best effects.

470 SPLASH SOME VINEGAR

The next time you're cooking meat or fish, add a splash of vinegar, which has been shown to help leach out the calcium, making your meal more nutritious and bone-healthy. It also works on green salads, so make sure you use a vinegar-based dressing.

471 GO BANANAS

Eating a banana a day can help keep bones healthy because they contain high levels of potassium. This is thought to equalize mineral levels in the blood, meaning the bones can hold on to their strength-building calcium supplies.

472 EAT AN APPLE A DAY

Apples are a good choice for a daily dose against osteoporosis because they contain boron, a trace element essential for healthy bones. It's found in pears, almonds, grapes, dates, hazelnuts and peanuts as well, but apples are a great source.

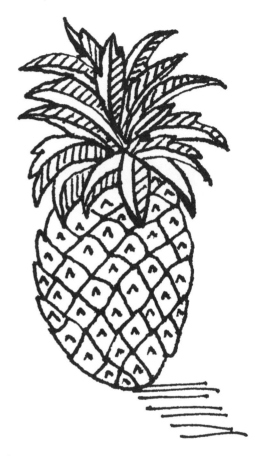

473 PICK A PINEAPPLE

Pineapple juice is a good option at breakfast time because it contains manganese, a deficiency linked to the development of osteoporosis. Manganese is also in oatmeal, nuts, cereals, spinach and black tea, but pineapple is a plentiful source.

474 GO FIG-URE

Figs are very high in calcium, so they're a great choice for bone health. Eat them with low-fat natural live (active culture) yogurt, which also contains high calcium levels, and make sure you stay well hydrated, as dehydration can affect your calcium uptake.

475 MAKE IT MILKY

Milk is the number one choice for bone health, and skimmed milk is the best of all because the calcium it contains is most easily accessible for your digestive system. Aim for 250 ml (8 fl oz) of milk a day to give you one third of your calcium allowance. If you don't like milk, salmon and sardines are other good sources, or try almond milk.

476 OJ AND MILK

Drink a glass of orange juice alongside your glass of milk. Chances are, they sit alongside each other in your fridge. Taking them together can be helpful too, because for your body to absorb calcium (from milk), it needs high levels of vitamin C (from orange juice). Perfect fridge-fellows!

477 SO SOY

Soya and tofu are thought to work as a bone strengthener because they contain soy isoflavones (phytoestrogens) that mimic the effect of oestrogens in the body, one of which is bone strength. Soya beans can be grown from pots in the garden, but need protecting with chicken wire.

478 USE YOGURT

Wherever possible, try to substitute low-fat natural live yogurt for cream, sour cream and crème fraîche in recipes. Yogurt is naturally high in calcium and even people who are lactose intolerant can usually eat it as the lactose is already broken down.

479 BE CHASTE

Chasteberry contains two powerful compounds which help to keep hormone levels in balance and therefore work in the same way as soy products to help bones stay strong and healthy.

480 OPEN SESAME

A handful of sesame seeds eaten every morning before breakfast could help the fight against osteoporosis – it is thought they contain plant oestrogens which can help prevent bone density loss.

RESTLESS LEGS

481 SIP TONIC WATER

There is some evidence that the quinine levels in tonic water could help reduce restless legs syndrome if drunk in the evening before bed. Try sipping a glass throughout the evening to see results.

482 GET HOTTER.

Sometimes a change from a hot temperature to a cold one, or vice versa, can help relieve restless legs. Try putting a heating pad or hot water bottle on your legs; alternatively, apply a cool compress to your legs, or dip your feet in cool water.

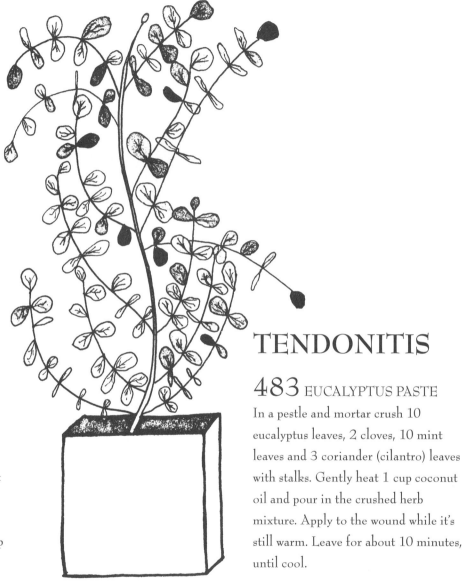

TENDONITIS

483 EUCALYPTUS PASTE

In a pestle and mortar crush 10 eucalyptus leaves, 2 cloves, 10 mint leaves and 3 coriander (cilantro) leaves with stalks. Gently heat 1 cup coconut oil and pour in the crushed herb mixture. Apply to the wound while it's still warm. Leave for about 10 minutes, until cool.

484 LOVE A LINIMENT

Make a liniment for tendonitis relief by mixing 2 tablespoons sesame seed or sunflower oil with 1 tablespoon turpentine. Apply directly to sore or injured tendons for immediate relief. An alternative recipe is ½ cup sunflower oil with 1 teaspoonful liquid camphor oil.

485 BANDAGE WITH GARLIC AND MUSTARD

Crush 2 to 3 cloves garlic and mix with 1 tablespoon mustard oil. Apply to the wound with a clean cloth. Then cover with a warm hand towel or cloth and leave for 10 to 15 minutes.

486 TURMERIC AND GINGER PASTE

Add 1 teaspoon turmeric powder to 1 teaspoon chopped fresh ginger root. Apply directly to the site of the injury and bandage securely. If there is a lot of swelling, add some rock salt to the paste as well. Leave for 10 to 15 minutes before rinsing off.

ACNE

487 OAT FACE PACK

Mix up natural oatmeal with some natural yogurt until a thick paste forms. Apply this mixture to your face, leave to dry, then wash off with warm water and pat dry. The yogurt will gently moisturize while the oatmeal helps reduce spots and redness. An alternative to this is to make up oatmeal with milk or water, then add some honey.

488 SAY HELLO TO ALOE

Aloe vera is a great plant for all skin irritation, especially on delicate skin like the face and neck. Boil a handful of chopped aloe leaves in 2 cups water, then strain to make a face wash. Or apply directly onto the areas you want to treat.

489 GET BERRY SMOOTH

Boil a handful of strawberry leaves (wild strawberry plants are often mistaken for weeds in gardens) or blackberry (bramble) leaves in 1 litre (1¾ pints) water. Allow to cool and apply to the face to relieve dryness, itching and irritation.

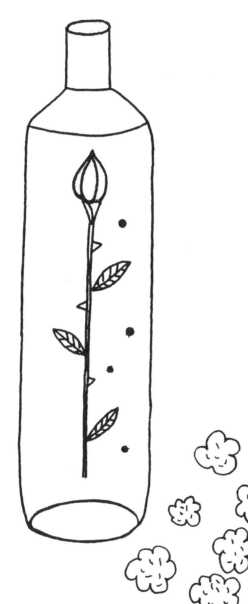

490 GET A WITCH CURE

When used as a topical spot cream, witch hazel is one of the best natural remedies as it contains natural antiseptic and antibacterial properties as well as being soothing, so it reduces redness as well.

491 TIME FOR TEA

Empty out two ordinary tea bags into a small saucepan and add about half the amount of dried basil. Simmer with 2 cups of water for about 10 minutes, then strain. Apply the liquid directly to breakouts with cotton wool.

492 GET ROSY CHEEKS

If you suffer from blemishes or acne, mix up equal amounts of rose water and lemon or lime juice and apply with clean cotton wool to thoroughly cleansed skin. Wait 15 minutes, then rinse off. The citrus is a natural astringent, while the rose water calms and soothes sore skin. For very dry skin, add a little milk as well.

493 ZAP ZITS WITH TOOTHPASTE

If you have very greasy skin, toothpaste is a good way to dry out spots as it helps dehydrate only the area it touches. Use it as a spot cream as soon as you feel pimples arising to dry them out and reduce swelling.

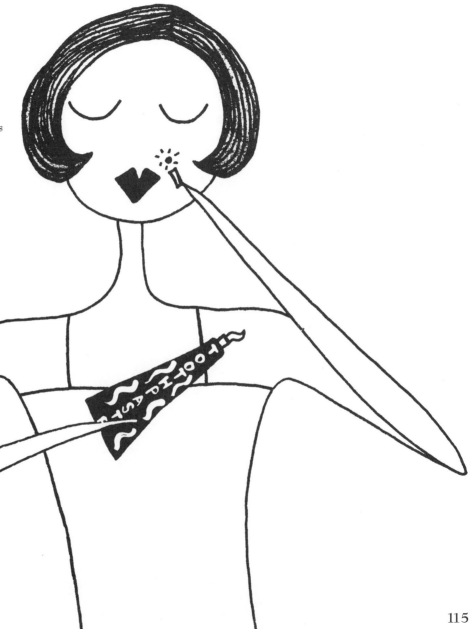

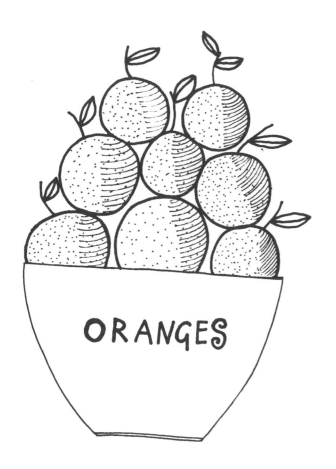

494 GRIND AN ORANGE

Don't throw away your orange peel next time you eat the fruit – grind up the peel in a pestle and mortar and use the resulting mush to treat acne spots on your face and body. Rinse off after 5 to 10 minutes.

495 SUGAR YOUR SKIN

Mix 1 tablespoon brown sugar (to exfoliate) with 3 tablespoons honey (to moisturize and calm angry skin) and add a pinch of cinnamon (to help reduce acne and spots). Use this as a mild face scrub and mask before bed.

496 GET GRATE SKIN

Apple and cucumber both contain skin-calming chemicals, so grate 1 tablespoon of each and mix together with an equal amount of honey. Apply as a face mask for 10 to 15 minutes before rinsing gently and patting dry.

497 SEASON YOUR MILK

Into 125 ml (4 fl oz) of milk grate at least 1 teaspoon grated fresh nutmeg. Use the solution to rinse acne-affected skin. Leave to dry and don't wash for a few hours, then rinse off and pat dry. Repeat as desired.

498 CLOVE AWAY SPOTS

Using milk infused with cloves or clove oil is a good facial wash for acne-prone skin, or try a different type of clove – peel a clove of garlic and rub it directly onto the spot to reduce inflammation, speed up healing and lessen scarring.

499 REDUCE SPOTS WITH TOMATO PURÉE

Tomatoes are thought to be very good for reducing spots due to acne as they alter the acidity of the skin surface, making infection less likely. Use tomato purée as a spot cream before bed (watch those white pillows!) to reduce spottiness.

500 APPLY TEA TREE

Applying tea tree oil can prevent spots becoming worse and help to dry up those already in existence. Apply directly to the affected area to help clear up congested skin.

501 GET ON YOUR NETTLE

Nettle might be a strange choice for reducing skin irritation, as it can cause stinging, but the leaves have anti-inflammatory properties when taken as tea. Make nettle tea by filling a teapot with leaves, pouring over boiling water and steeping for 5 to 10 minutes, then drink as desired. Be sure to wear gloves when handling uncooked nettle leaves.

502 SHRINK SPOTS WITH PEPPERMINT

Peppermint is a great anti-acne herb because it contains menthol, which is known to help reduce swelling, but you could use spearmint as well. Simply crush some leaves and apply the leaves and their juice as a facepack for 5 to 10 minutes before rinsing and patting dry.

503 MAKE IT MANUKA

Manuka honey – which is made by bees in New Zealand with the pollen from the tea tree plant – has amazing antibacterial properties, making it a great anti-blemish choice. Use it as a face mask, facial wash or apply directly as a leave-on cream.

504 BLITZ BOILS WITH PEROXIDE AND HONEY

Wash the infected area with soap and water, apply a drop of hydrogen peroxide and allow to dry. Cover the boil with honey and repeat several times the first day. The next day, apply a warm wet cloth to bring up the head and continue applying peroxide and honey until it disappears.

SCARS & SUN SPOTS

505 ONIONS AND VINEGAR

Finely chop a onion and use a muslin or strainer to extract the juice, or use a juicer. Mix one part of this onion juice with one part of cider vinegar and apply the formulation directly to scarred or discoloured areas of skin.

506 RUB WITH POTATO

Rubbing a slice of potato on your skin could help reduce scarring and discolouration because it acts as a very mild natural bleach. Lemon juice acts in the same way, but be careful around your eyes.

507 GET HIP WITH ROSE

Rosehip can help heal scarring and reverse skin discolouration. Simply cut a rosehip in half and wipe over the scar, or make a rosehip tea to use as a refreshing facial rinse following cleansing.

508 CHOOSE COCONUT

Coconut milk is a good choice for scars – use either the milk or a coconut oil to massage into scars to help reduce the appearance of the white keloid tissue and encourage facial skin to become more even in tone.

509 VICTORY WITH VITAMINS

Vitamin E is simply the most powerful anti-scar remedy, as even on old scars a direct application can lead to the scar reducing dramatically – and in some cases disappearing altogether – within a few weeks. Apply oil directly to the scar, or open a vitamin E capsule and apply the oil.

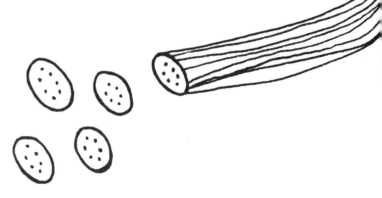

510 CURE WITH CUCUMBER SLICES

Applying fresh cucumber juice can help reduce scarring as it maintains the right fluid balance in the skin, which helps it heal more effectively. Juice a cucumber and use the liquid as a lotion; alternatively, lie still with fresh cucumber slices over affected areas.

511 PICK PAPAYA

The inside of papaya skin can be used to help reduce scarring as it contains enzymes and compounds which help the skin heal itself naturally. Wipe the inside of a papaya skin over your face, leave for an hour and wash off with warm water. This will also help blemishes.

512 STICK ON SOME HONEY

If you are worried about scarring, try smearing honey over the affected area – it is thought to help the skin cells bind together, reducing the appearance of scars by speeding up the healing process.

513 MAKE A MINT

Crush a handful of mint leaves and wrap them in a piece of muslin (cheesecloth). Then squeeze and roll to extract the juice. Wipe the bag over your face using gentle circular movements. Repeat daily to help reduce scarring.

514 SANDALWOOD AND ROSE PASTE

Sandalwood can help scars left by acne or other skin conditions. Make a paste by rubbing a sandalwood stick on a wooden board with some rose water, then use as a facepack before rinsing. Alternatively use a few drops of sandalwood essential oil with rose water.

STRETCHMARKS

515 EAT YOUR SEEDS

Zinc is very important for the healing of stretchmarks, particularly those caused by pregnancy. Get yours from nuts, seeds and seafood.

516 MASSAGE AWAY MARKS

Using a base of almond oil, add a few drops each of lavender and camomile essential oils. Massage the oil onto the stretchmarks once or twice a day to help reduce their appearance.

517 GO 100%

Natural cocoa butter contains really high levels of vitamin E, so it's great for helping dry skin and reducing stretch marks and scarring. Invest in a 100% cocoa butter stick and you can rub it directly onto skin or cut off a chunk and use in the bath as oil.

518 SOAP IT ON

Using a natural vitamin E soap can help reduce stretchmarks if added to the bath – simply use in your tub with a few drops of lavender and camomile essential oils to help heal and moisturize.

519 JUICE UP A VITAMIN RUB

Place 1 cup olive oil, ½ cup aloe vera gel, and the liquid from 10 vitamin E capsules and 6 vitamin A capsules in a blender. Whizz together and store in the fridge in a covered jar. Use once or twice daily to massage into affected areas.

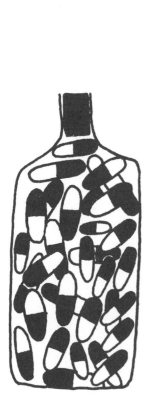
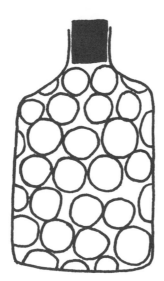

ROSACEA

520 GO GREEN

Green tea cream is thought to have a calming and regenerating effect on rosacea – make your own using regular aqueous cream mixed with strong green tea, or try chrysanthemum flowers instead to flavour your cream.

521 WIPE ON LIQUORICE

Liquorice tea has an anti-redness effect on skin – rinse daily with strong liquorice tea to help see effects, or use morning and night if your rosacea is very bad.

522 AN APPLE A DAY

Apple cider vinegar is a good home remedy for rosacea when drunk with water as it is reputed to help regulate the balance of good and bad bacteria in the stomach, which is thought to be linked to rosacea. Dilute 1 teaspoon vinegar in 125 ml (4 fl oz) water and drink daily.

523 BREW A FENUGREEK TEA

Drink 2 to 3 cups of fenugreek tea a day – made from the seeds or fresh leaves – to help reduce rosacea; it can also treat acne and acne scarring.

WRINKLES

524 GET EGGY

The skin under your eyes is prone to dryness and can wrinkle – help it retain moisture using egg whites. Simply apply them to the area under your eyes, allow to dry and then rinse off with warm water. Or use castor oil instead if you don't like eggs.

525 OIL THEM AWAY

Mix up an anti-wrinkle treatment with ½ cup comfrey tea, ½ cup witch hazel and 10 drops patchouli essential oil. Store in a clean bottle and apply to wrinkles every night before bed to help firm your skin.

526 GO FOR GLYCERINE

Mix 1 tablespoon each of glycerine and rose water, then add a few drops of lime juice. Apply to the face for an instant moisturizing treat. Leave for 15 to 20 minutes before rinsing off. Finish by drinking a glass of water to help hydrate skin.

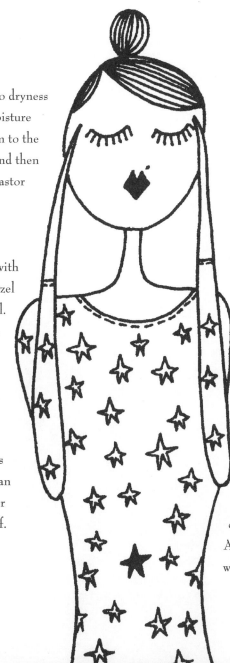

527 MASSAGE WRINKLES

To help slow down the ageing process and prevent more wrinkles appearing, gently massage coconut oil into wrinkles every night. Alternatively make a paste of turmeric with sugar and water and massage in.

528 BE FINE WITH FLAX

Flaxseed oil is a great choice for getting rid of wrinkles
– take 1 tablespoon four times a day (it might take a
few days to build up to four, so start with twice a day
and build up slowly to avoid diarrhoea).

529 BANANA AND HONEY MASK

Mash up 1 banana and mix it with 1 tablespoon
each of honey and yogurt. Apply to the face for
20 minutes, then rinse off. This combination of
ingredients gives you a great calcium, magnesium and
potassium boost, which helps skin regeneration.

530 MAKE UP AN ANTI-WRINKLE MASK

Mix together 2 tablespoons plain yogurt,
½ tablespoon honey and ½ tablespoon lemon
juice. Add the liquid from 3 vitamin E capsules.
Apply to the face using a cotton ball. Leave
for 10 minutes before rinsing off.

531 GRAB A GRAPE

Cut a couple of grapes in half and rub over freshly
washed skin to help give it a dose of antioxidants.
Allow to dry for 20 minutes, then rinse off to
help reduce fine wrinkles. This also works with
fresh pineapple flesh.

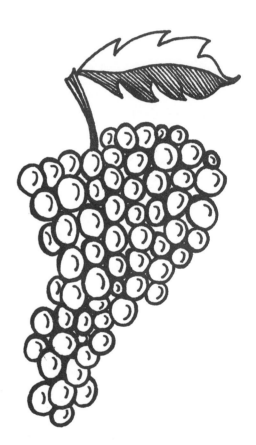

DRY SKIN

532 GET YOUR OATS

Add a cup of instant oatmeal to your warm bath –
they are packed with vitamin E, which is essential
for healthy skin and prevents dryness. Rub dry
hands with oatmeal instead of soap to help clean
without drying.

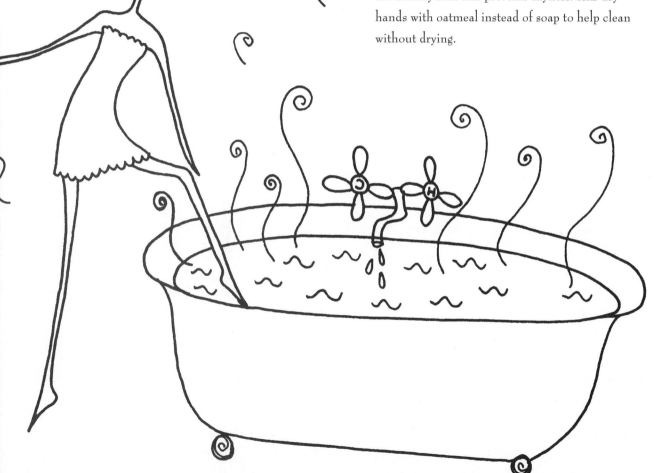

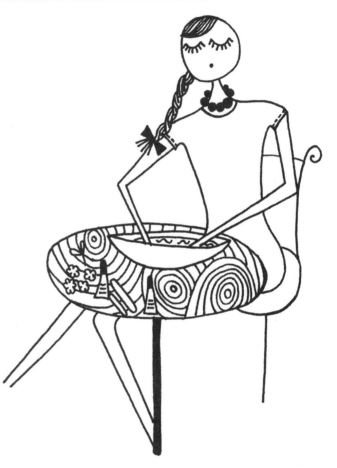

533 GET CORNY

Cornflour (cornstarch) is a good way to help relieve
dry skin – sprinkle a handful in your bath or use
bicarbonate of soda (baking soda) instead, which is
known to help dry skin and reduce itching.

534 EXFOLIATE WITH SALT

Any type of salt is a good way to exfoliate dry skin
away, as it helps to reduce dryness and itching and
boosts circulation. Pour a cupful into your bath
and use to rub over the skin (in the direction
of the heart) for several minutes.

535 OIL YOURSELF

Coat your skin in vegetable oil to help
reduce itching and add natural moisture.
Olive, almond and sesame oils are good choices.
Cover yourself and lie on a towel to soak up
excess moisture.

536 HEAL YOUR HANDS

If your hands are chapped and sore, soak them
in milk once a day. The lactic acid in milk will
moisturize your skin. Alternatively, mix a few drops
glycerine with a few drops lemon essential oil and
massage the mixture into the hands at bedtime.

OILY SKIN

537 AN EGG-YOLK CURE

Egg yolk is a good way to reduce blemishes because it absorbs oil. Apply a lightly whisked egg yolk to oily spots on your face with a cotton ball, leave for 10 minutes, then rinse off with warm water. Lemon juice exerts a similar effect if applied in an equal dilution with water.

538 SCRUB IT CLEAN

Adding ½ teaspoon bicarbonate of soda (baking soda) to your usual face wash or soap gives it a gentle abrasive quality, which helps reduce oil on troublesome areas of skin. Concentrate on the nose and chin, which are traditional oily spots.

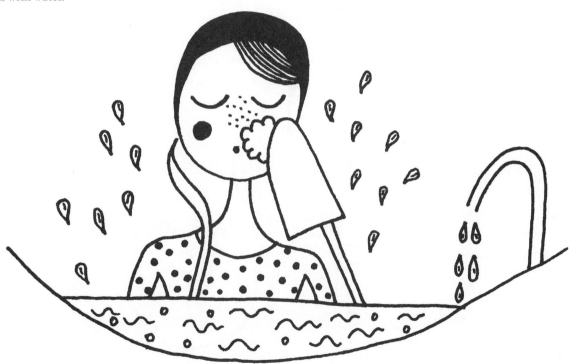

539 FLOUR IT AWAY

Cornflour (cornstarch) can be used on skin to help dry oily patches. Mix 1 tablespoon cornstarch with a little warm water to make a paste. Rub onto the face with circular motions, then allow to dry for 5 to 10 minutes. Rinse with cold water. Repeat once a day.

540 SPRAY WITH SALT AND VINEGAR

Salt can help to dry the skin when used mixed with water as a homemade facial spritz, or try using vinegar applied neat to the skin before bed as a natural exfoliator. If your skin is really prone to oiliness in the summer, make ice cubes from vinegar and use them to massage into facial skin.

541 STAY SWEET

A combination of ground almonds and honey works well as a gentle facial scrub for removing oil and dead skin cells without causing trauma to the skin surface. Mix equal amounts and blend to form a paste, then massage into skin with a warm cloth and rinse with cool water.

542 GET A FRUIT BOOST

Certain citrus fruits not only refresh the skin and add vitamins but also help reduce oils naturally. Mix up equal amounts of lime juice and cucumber juice and apply to skin. Leave for 5 minutes before rinsing off.

543 APPLE AND OATMEAL MASK

Mix together ½ cup oatmeal, 1 egg white and 1 tablespoon lemon juice. Add ½ cup grated or mashed peeled apple to the oatmeal mixture. Smooth the paste onto your face, leave for 15 minutes, then rinse off with cool water.

ECZEMA

544 GET DIRTY

Mud packs are a good choice for eczema as they contain high levels of nutrients as well as beneficial bacteria that can reduce redness and infection. Mix up a paste with water and ordinary garden mud, smear onto the affected area and leave for 5 to 10 minutes before rinsing off.

545 REDUCE ITCHING WITH SANDALWOOD

Sandalwood is a good choice for eczema as it moisturizes without putting undue stress on the delicate skin underlayers. Mix up equal amounts of sandalwood powder and liquid camphor and smear directly onto affected areas.

546 MAKE A FLOWER SOAP

Make your own anti-eczema soap by grating a large block of olive or vegetable soap into a small saucepan. Add 1 tablespoon oatmeal, a handful each camomile flowers and rose petals, and a few drops rose and camomile essential oils. Heat gently, mixing well, then pour into greaseproof (wax) paper set inside a mould. When cool, turn out and use as body soap.

547 GET WET

One of the best treatments for eczema is simple water. Simply use a cold wet compress on affected areas to help the skin regulate its moisture levels and reduce eczema symptoms.

548 RUB IT AWAY WITH NUTMEG

Rub a whole nutmeg against a smooth stone, or grate with a very fine grater, then add enough water to form a smooth paste. Apply to the eczema areas to help reduce the severity of an attack. You could also substitute mustard powder, frankincense or turmeric for the nutmeg. Always test an area on non-affected skin first.

549 CRUSH A PAPAYA CURE

Remove the round black seeds from inside a papaya. Wash and dry them and then crush in a liquidizer or pestle and mortar. Mix the crushed papaya seeds with a small amount of papaya juice and apply to the skin for 10 to 15 minutes.

550 GET OILY

Oils are a great choice for helping to reduce eczema symptoms as they stick around on the skin, so they carry on adding moisture for longer than lotions. Use coconut oil, shea butter or cocoa butter for best results.

551 BATHE IN MILK

If you suffer from eczema all over your body, try bathing in milk. Instead of filling a bath, which would be very expensive and wasteful, use a bowl and give yourself a milky sponge bath. Try to leave the milk on the skin for 10 minutes before showering off. Alternatively, add 1 cup of milk powder to your usual soak.

552 SOOTHE SKIN WITH HEMPSEED OIL

Naturally moisturizing and with the ability to penetrate deep into the skin, hempseed oil can relieve itchy inflamed skin. Apply direct to the affected area or take 1 teaspoon hempseed oil three times a day.

DERMATITIS & RASHES

553 DIP A TEA BAG

To soothe inflamed skin, dip a camomile tea bag in warm water and hold it onto the sore area of skin for a few minutes before patting dry. Reheat and repeat as needed.

554 RINSE WITH BLUEBERRIES

Blueberries and blueberry leaves contain high levels of antioxidants, which can help reduce swelling and boost skin healing. Mash them up and apply directly to skin as a mask. Leave for 10 minutes before rinsing off.

555 GET SWEET

Mix equal parts of apple cider vinegar with lemon juice and dab the solution onto the affected areas. Add a thin layer of honey on top to help seal in the healing effects. Rinse off after 5 to 10 minutes and moisturize your skin with a natural oil such as olive or almond.

556 TAKE IT FROM TREE

Tea tree oil is a good choice to use on dermatitis that has broken the skin, as it not only helps heal but also prevents infection from developing. Dilute with a light vegetable oil if your skin is very sore or weeping and dab on.

557 PICK UP POTASSIUM

Potassium is essential for healthy skin and if you suffer bouts of dermatitis you may be deficient. Get your source from avocado, apricots, banana, beans, parsley, peaches, wheatgerm, carrots, dried fruits and soyabeans.

558 A WITCHY SOLUTION

Witch hazel can help heal up eczema and dermatitis if used on sore skin as soon as it starts to develop. Mix with olive or almond oil so your skin is moisturized too, and apply three to five times a day as required.

559 MAKE MINE A BLOODY MARY

Tomato juice is thought to help cure eczema and dermatitis by regulating the acidity level of the skin and providing the antioxidant vitamins and minerals needed for healing.

PSORIASIS

560 WRAP IT UP

Wrapping up psoriasis patches with cling film (plastic wrap) is a good way to help lesions disappear. You can use it to cover medications or simply the lesions themselves. Leave it on for up to an hour but don't let the skin go soggy.

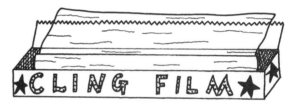

561 GET WARM

Olive oil is a good cure for psoriasis if warmed gently and used to massage affected areas. Don't rinse off afterwards – just allow to soak naturally into the skin.

562 BATHE IN SALTS

Adding ½ cup of Epsom salts, bicarbonate of soda (baking soda) or mineral oil to your bath can all help psoriasis by soothing skin, reducing itching and regulating moisture. Alternatively, add a glass of milk and 1 tablespoon olive oil to your bathwater to boost moisture.

CELLULITE

563 GRAB SOME COFFEE GROUNDS

The caffeine in coffee has long been believed to help reduce cellulite if used as a scrub – simply grab a handful of wet coffee grounds and use them to vigorously massage affected areas. Do this every morning or evening for two weeks to see results.

564 WRAP IT UP

Exfoliate your skin well, then dry and massage with almond or olive oil to which you have added a few drops of orange essential oil. Wrap snugly in cellophane and leave for 30 minutes to soak in.

565 FIND SOME FENNEL

Fennel seeds are a good choice for beating cellulite as they help the body break fat deposits down. Eat a spoonful of fennel seeds once a day with a glass of water for best results.

566 THYME FOR A CHANGE

Give your body a double dose of thyme by drinking thyme tea and infusing some oil to massage cellulite daily. Do this for a week and you should see results begin to show.

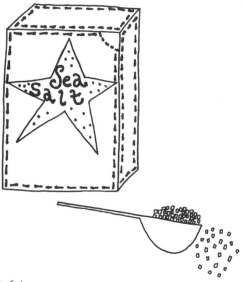

567 BATHE IN SALT

Salt bathing is a good way to reduce cellulite, especially if you use it to massage and exfoliate affected areas at the same time. Sea salt contains the best mixture of minerals.

568 MAKE A GIN-BATH BLEND

To a bath add a few drops of each of the following essential oils: grapefruit, geranium, fennel, thyme and lavender, then add a shot of gin. Soak for 10 minutes, then use a loofah or body brush to massage over your cellulite in upward strokes (towards the heart) for 20 minutes. When you've finished, shower off with a cold blast.

WARTS & VERRUCAS

569 TAPE IT UP

One of the best ways to get rid of warts is to apply heavy-duty duct tape over it. Change the tape regularly and leave until the wart disappears (usually within a month, as it suffocates).

570 SLICE YOUR GARLIC

A good remedy for warts is to slice a clove of garlic and place it over the wart or verruca, then put a plaster (bandaid) over the top to hold it in place. Only leave for an hour at a time, though, as garlic is potent.

571 TRICKLE ON TEA TREE

Simply add a drop or two of tea tree oil to the top of the wart or verruca three times a day and you should begin to see it shrinking and changing colour within three days; it should disappear within three weeks.

572 SOAK A PENNY

Soak a copper penny in vinegar until the mixture turns green and then bathe your wart or verruca in vinegar every night before bed. The copper ions are thought to help reduce wart growth.

573 PICK A POTATO

Cut a piece of raw potato to the same size as the wart, then secure it over the top of the wart with tape or a plaster (bandaid). Change regularly, and simply keep repeating until the wart disappears.

574 MILK A DANDELION

Take a dandelion flower in bloom, cut off the stem at the bottom and squeeze out the white fluid. Use this to cover the wart three times a day, letting it dry naturally.

575 MAKE A LEEK POULTICE

Houseleek is a common garden plant that is related to aloe and has amazing anti-wart properties. Simply cut a houseleek leaf in half and press the flesh and juice onto the wart. Hold in place with tape and change morning and evening.

576 USE A BANANA RUB

Peel a banana and use the inside of the skin to rub on the wart or verruca several times a day until the wart disappears. It is thought the high levels of potassium (more concentrated in the skin) prevent the wart from growing.

THINNING HAIR & HAIR LOSS

577 VOLUMIZE HAIR NATURALLY

For natural body-building, mix Epsom salts with conditioner, warm in a saucepan or microwave bowl and work the mixture through the hair, leaving for 20 minutes before rinsing.

578 ROSEMARY AND SAGE SHAMPOO

Both rosemary and sage are natural astringents and rosemary has the added benefit of being a skin toner. Together they stimulate hair follicles and condition the scalp. To use, simmer equal amounts of fresh rosemary and sage in a water for 10 minutes. Then strain the loose herbs from the liquid and use the liquid to wash your hair. Repeat daily.

579 STIMULATE WITH MASSAGE

Use a blend of 6 drops each lavender and bay essential oils in a base of 125 ml (4 fl oz) of either almond or sesame oil. Massage into the scalp and leave for 20 minutes. Massaging the scalp every day can encourage blood flow to the hair follicles and help stimulate some hair growth.

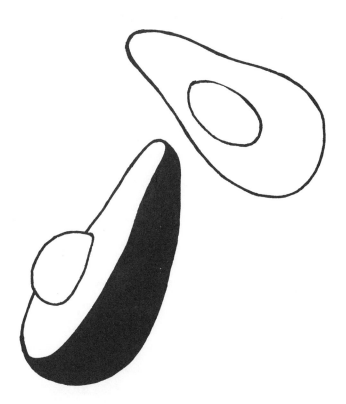

580 SPEED HAIR GROWTH WITH AVOCADO

To encourage hair growth, mash the fruit of an avocado and apply the paste to your head and scalp. Wrap up, leave overnight and wash as usual the next morning. This also helps the skin to regenerate, although only use it for 20 minutes.

DANDRUFF

581 RINSE WITH VINEGAR

Rinsing your scalp with apple cider vinegar can help slough off dead skin cells and recondition dry and flaking scalps. You can also use milk or cucumber juice that has been infused with a fresh garlic clove.

582 SOAK IN EPSOM

Epsom salts may be used to soak up excess oil from your hair – add a few tablespoons to your usual shampoo and massage into dry hair and scalp. Rinse with water. Follow with a rinse of lemon juice or apple cider vinegar, leave for 5 minutes and rinse thoroughly.

583 USE YUCCA FOR DANDRUFF AND ITCHING

The Mojave yucca (*Yucca schidigera*) was used by Native Americans to fight dandruff and hair loss. It contains a high concentration of saponins, a natural detergent, and has anti-inflammatory properties. To use, take a piece of yucca root (which includes the trunk of the plant) and peel off the brown outer layer. Pound the root with a mallet, then run it under water – it will lather up like a soap. Use to wash the hair and rinse well.

584 MAKE A FENUGREEK AND LEMON PASTE

Soak 2 tablespoons fenugreek seeds overnight in water, then drain. Use a liquidizer, coffee grinder or mortar and pestle to grind the seeds into a fine paste with a little lemon or lime juice. Apply to scalp, leave overnight and shampoo out in the morning.

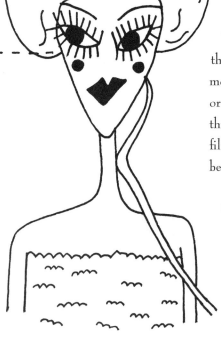

DRY HAIR & SCALP

585 MAKE A MAYONNAISE MASK

For a super-moisturizing treat, beat 2 eggs with 2 tablespoons olive oil and 2 tablespoons vinegar. Massage into the hair, cover with a shower cap or cling film (plastic wrap), and leave for 30 minutes. Shampoo and condition as usual. You can also use shop-bought mayonnaise, if you prefer.

586 HAVE A HOT-OIL SOAK

The oil helps rehydrate the hair shaft and the heat helps the hair and scalp absorb moisture. Gently heat ¼ cup olive, coconut or almond oil, then massage in well, working through the hair shaft. Cover with cling film (plastic wrap) and leave for 20 minutes before shampooing as usual.

587 SOOTHE BRITTLE HAIR WITH COCONUT MILK

Add 2 tablespoons gram flour to 1 cup coconut milk and gently massage into the scalp. Leave for 5 to 10 minutes, then rinse.

588 RUB IN ALOE

Aloe vera gel helps moisturize dry hair and prevents weakness. Remove some of the gel from a fresh plant leaf and rub into the scalp. Leave for 10 to 15 minutes, then rinse thoroughly. Shampoo, if required.

HAIR REMOVAL

589 GOODBYE UNWANTED FACIAL HAIR

Mix together a paste of 3 teaspoons gram flour and 1 teaspoon powdered turmeric with a little water and apply to the face. Allow to dry, then gently rub off using circular motions.

590 DEPILATE WITH SUGAR

Mix 1 cup granulated sugar with the juice of ½ lemon and ¼ cup honey. Set over a very low heat until it bubbles and turns a rich amber. Allow to cool slightly. Dust your legs with cornflour (cornstarch) and spread a thin layer of the warm mixture on each leg in the direction of hair growth. Cover with a strip of cotton fabric, pressing down, then pull the strip off from one end in the opposite direction of hair growth.

BODY ODOUR

591 WIPE SMELLS AWAY

Soak a cotton ball in white wine or cider vinegar and wipe the whole of your underarm area. The smell of vinegar will disappear after a few minutes and your underarms will stay fresh for much longer.

592 SOAK IN TOMATO

Add a few cups of tomato juice to your bath and soak for around 15 minutes. Tomato helps restore the skin's natural pH levels, which reduce smell-producing bacteria.

593 SMELL GRATE!

Grate a raw turnip and squeeze the juice from the grated pieces, or use a juicer to extract pure turnip juice, then wipe the liquid under the arms.

594 GET WHEATY

Drink a glass of water every morning along with 30 ml (1½ fl oz) wheatgrass juice or a 500 mg tablet. It is thought that the chlorophyll in the wheatgrass helps reduce or even prevent body odour. Keep drinking water throughout the day as dehydration can also contribute. Available in health food stores as fresh produce, tablets, frozen juice and powder, wheatgrass can also be easily grown at home and juiced.

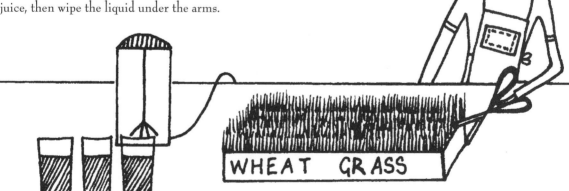

WHEAT GRASS

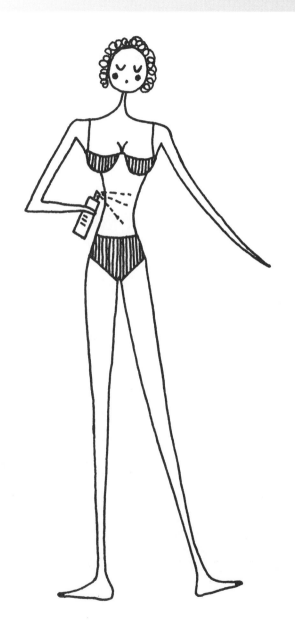

595 MAKE YOUR OWN DEODORANT

Extract the juice from approximately 20 radishes and add 20 drops of liquid glycerine (available from most pharmacies). Store in the fridge and use in a spray bottle or dab onto underarms.

596 HAVE A MINT BATH

Mint is another great herb for soaking up body odour smells to leave you smelling fresh and clean. Boil up a handful of fresh mint leaves, strain and add the liquid to your bath.

597 BE A POTATO HEAD

Raw potato can be used if you've run out of deodorant – simply slice a potato in half and rub the cut halves on your underarms to reduce smells and prevent body odour appearing for several hours.

598 SPRAY IT AWAY

Tea tree is a great deodorizer as well as antibacterial, so it gets rid of odour-producing bacteria. Mix 15 to 20 drops of the essential oil in around 50 ml (2 fl oz) water and decant into a spray bottle to apply as topical deodorant, or dab on with cotton wool balls.

599 BAKE IT AWAY

Bicarbonate of soda (baking soda) can be used to help 'soak up' smells and stop new ones appearing. Apply directly to your armpits to reduce odour or mix with lemon for a really fresh smell.

600 ROSE TO THE OCCASION

To help prevent body odour, add a few drops of rose essential oil or rose water to your bath. This helps give your skin a freshness that lasts all day and will help reduce body odours.

601 EAT YOUR RADISHES

Red radishes in the diet are a great way of cutting down on body odour – try to eat them several times a week (raw in salads) and particularly if you are having 'smelly' foods like curry or strong flavours.

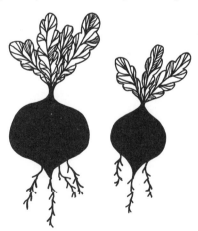

SMELLY FEET

602 SOAK IN VINEGAR

The best way to stop feet from smelling is to soak them for 10 minutes in a basin of one part vinegar to two parts warm water. Magic!

603 HAVE A CUP OF TEA

For smelly feet, try soaking twice a day in strong tea (without the milk!). Tea contains tannin, which is a powerful drying agent that will help stop your feet sweating as much and therefore reduce smells.

604 BATHE IN ROCK SALT

For a great anti-odour foot soak, use rock salt dissolved in warm water. The salt helps neutralize nasty smells and acts as an anti-inflammatory to help stop inflammation and odour production.

605 A SOCK-FULL OF OATS

To soak up sweat in your socks and reduce the smell of sweaty feet, add a handful of bran or oats to your socks – it might be a strange sensation to start with, but it will soak up the sweat, leaving your feet odour-free.

606 HAVE A FOOT BATH

Bicarbonate of soda (baking powder) is a great way to help stop your feet from smelling as it increases the acidity of your foot's surface and stops odour being produced. Add 1 tablespoon to a footbath of water and soak for 15 minutes. Alternatively, sprinkle bicarb in tennis shoes, socks, boots and slippers to eliminate odour.

607 BE SAGE

Try sprinkling dried, crushed sage leaves in your shoes to help your feet dry and reduce perspiration.

608 WATCH WHAT YOU EAT

If you are prone to smelly feet, try to reduce the amount of strong-smelling foods like garlic, chilli and highly spiced foods in your diet as these may contribute to your foot-odour problem. Choose fragrant, mild foods like lemon and ginger instead.

609 SOAK IN TEA TREE

Tea tree oil isn't just a good antiseptic, it's also great for getting rid of odours and perspiration. Add 10 to 15 drops to a basin of warm water and soak for 15 minutes every day to reduce smell.

SORE & ACHING FEET

610 SCATTER YOUR BEANS

For a great exercise to stimulate tired feet and help strengthen foot muscles, scatter some dried beans on the floor and spend a few minutes each day trying to pick them up with your toes. It will give your feet a great workout.

611 GO HOT AND COLD

The best type of foot soak to help sore and aching feet is to alternate between two basins of water, one warm and one cool, because that helps calm the nerves. Avoid water that is too extreme in temperature as this could actually cause the feet to hurt more.

612 TURN UP A TURNIP

Peel a large turnip and boil it until it's soft, for about 10 minutes. Spread the soft pulp on two handkerchiefs or face cloths and apply one to each foot, wrapping round to secure. Elevate your feet and relax for 15 to 30 minutes before washing off.

613 HAVE AN EPSOM BATH

For a most relaxing and pain-reducing foot soak, add Epsom salts to your foot soak or bath, and try to sit for a short time afterwards with your feet elevated to reduce inflammation.

614 ICE YOUR FEET

If your feet are tired from a day of over-use (but not if you suffer arthritis or other foot problems), give them a dose of instant relief using a pack of frozen peas wrapped in a teatowel.

615 FOOT SOAK WITH TEA

Make yourself a relaxing foot soak with 1 cup cider vinegar, 2 tablespoons Epsom salts and 2 cups peppermint or camomile tea (or a mixture of the two, if you prefer). Soak for at least 10 minutes.

616 BE A LEMON

For extra relief from aching, tired feet, massage with lemon juice after soaking, then rinse in cool water and pat dry.

CORNS & CALLOUSES

617 MAKE AN ONION COMPRESS

For corns, soak a slice of onion in vinegar for 4 hours, then place it over the corn and secure in place with a bandage or strip of fabric. Cover with a sock and leave overnight.

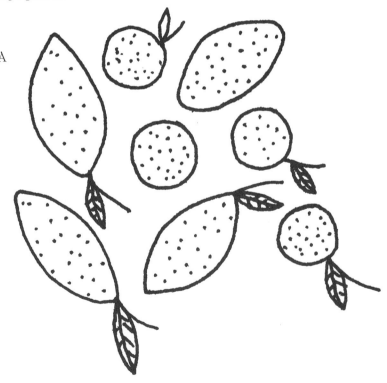

618 REDUCE PAIN WITH A FRUIT POULTICE

The enzymes in fresh lemon and pineapple are thought to help reduce the pain of corns. Place the inside of the peel over the corn, with the fruit side touching your corn, and secure in place firmly overnight with a bandage or strip of fabric. Papaya pulp or peel is thought to work in the same way.

619 GET A TEATIME CURE

Whenever you make yourself a cup of tea at home, save the tea bag and place it over your corn for 20 minutes to help reduce the severity. A few times a day should start to make a difference in no time at all.

620 EASE CORNS WITH BREWER'S YEAST

Make a paste using 1 teaspoon brewer's yeast and a few drops lemon juice, then apply directly to the corn and cover well with a bandage. Replace morning and evening.

621 FILE IT AWAY

If you've used a home remedy overnight on your corn or callous, make sure you spend a few minutes in the morning filing it away – a few drops of olive oil can help soften the skin beforehand.

COLD FEET

622 STIMULATE CIRCULATION WITH PEPPER

Use an old ski remedy and sprinkle some black pepper or cayenne pepper into your socks before you put them on, or rub the pepper directly on the soles to help circulation and keep the feet warm. If you use cayenne pepper, be prepared for both feet and socks to turn red!

623 DAMP SALT RUB

Stimulate the circulation in your cold feet by soaking them in a basin of warm water with ½ cup of salt dissolved in it for 15 minutes. Afterwards, massage with damp salt.

624 STEP IN PLACE

A great way to help your feet regain their warmth if they're cold is to stand on your toes for 30 seconds, then come back down to your heels. Repeat several times to help stimulate blood flow and warm them up.

ATHLETE'S FOOT

625 EXPOSE TO SUNSHINE

Try to expose your feet to sunlight for at least
1 hour every day. Natural sunlight kills the fungus
that causes athlete's foot, so getting out and about
is a great natural remedy.

626 STOP FUNGUS WITH ALCOHOL

At night, apply some surgical spirit (rubbing alcohol)
to your feet. After they have dried, follow with a
sprinkling of unscented talcum powder. This 'chokes'
the fungus, stopping it from spreading.

627 CURE WITH GARLIC

Crush a clove of garlic, apply to the area affected with
athlete's foot, and leave for 30 minutes. Rinse with warm
water. Repeat once a day to help beat athlete's foot. If the
garlic burns your skin, remove and rinse immediately.
You can try again after 24 hours with diluted garlic juice.

628 GINGER FOOT SOAK

Ginger has antifungal properties, so is a great
treatment for athlete's foot. Infuse hot water with
fresh ginger root, allow to cool and then use as
a foot soak for 15 minutes twice a day.

629 MAKE IT PLAIN SAILING

Plain old cornflour (cornstarch) makes an excellent
anti-athlete's foot dusting powder. Use it to dust
clean feet and in socks.

630 FEET TO A TEA

Applying tea tree oil two or three times a day directly
to the affected area can not only help to banish
athlete's foot but stop it from returning. Tea tree has
very potent antifungal properties. If the itching is
very severe, combine tea tree oil with aloe vera gel
as an ointment or spray.

631 GET TOUCHY-FEELY

Using grapefruit seed
oil to massage your feet
twice daily can help to
reduce athlete's foot as
the extract is an anti-
fungal. Make your own
foot massage oil using
grapefruit seed extract, a
carrier oil such as almond
oil and a few drops of tea
tree essential oil.

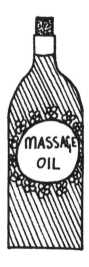

BUNIONS

632 CHOOSE CAMOMILE

Camomile can help reduce the pain and swelling of bunions and rebalance the fluid distribution. Every night thoroughly dampen a camomile tea bag with hot water, then use it to gently massage the joint for 5 to 10 minutes.

633 GIVE BUNIONS THE COLD SHOULDER

Ice away the pain of swollen bunions using a cold compress – apply frozen peas or ice wrapped in a towel onto the area for 10 to 15 minutes to alleviate that burning, swollen feeling.

634 USE YOUR WINE CORKS

Cork is a great way to help space your toes overnight if you suffer from bunions. Keep the corks from your wine bottles and cut them to a comfortable size to space between your big and first toes.

635 REDUCE SWELLING WITH EPSOM

To reduce the pain and swelling of bunions, soak them in very warm water into which you have dissolved Epsom salts. This will reduce the swelling of the joint and thus reduce the pain.

636 MASSAGE WITH COCONUT OIL

Every night before bed, massage your feet for 5 to 10 minutes using warm coconut oil – concentrate on the bunion area and massage to the bottom rather than from side to side. Following the massage, wear a pair of warm socks overnight to maximize the benefits.

TOENAIL FUNGUS

637 BE CORNY

Cover the bottom of a basin or footbath with yellow or white cornmeal and add just enough warm water to cover it. Let it stand for 30 minutes, then soak your feet in the solution for an hour. Repeat weekly.

638 RUB IT AWAY

Rub Vicks VapoRub (or make a homemade version using olive oil with a few drops each of peppermint and eucalyptus essential oils) onto your feet every night and cover with socks immediately. Repeat every night until the fungus disappears (this could take six to eight weeks).

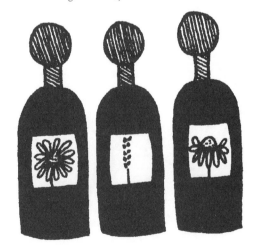

DRY EYES

639 APPLY A WARM COMPRESS

The best way to help dry eyes is to use a warm compress, which will gently encourage them to re-moisturize. Soak a small clean towel in warm water, wring it out and then lie down and apply the compress to your eyes for a few minutes until the dryness has eased.

640 TAKE TAMARIND

For dry eyes, soak tamarind seeds in water for several hours and then take 2 to 3 teaspoons of the resulting liquid daily to help cure dry eyes.

641 RELY ON ROSE

You should be very careful what you put into your eyes, but rose water can be used as a gentle, moisturizing eye-drop formula and is especially good for tired or red eyes.

POOR VISION

642 MIX UP A CARROT COCKTAIL

A 'good vision' cocktail can be easily made from the contents of your fridge. Combine 200 ml (7 fl oz) carrot juice, 150 ml (¼ pint) celery juice, 75 ml (3 fl oz) chicory or endive juice and 75 ml (3 fl oz) parsley juice. Drink daily to help combat eye problems.

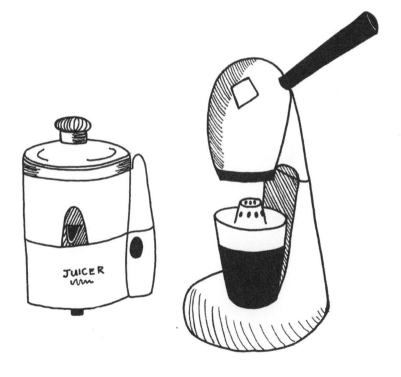

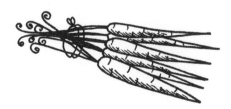

643 'A' IS FOR GOOD VISION

Vitamin A is essential for maintaining good vision. To help prevent eye problems, make sure your diet contains lots of foods rich in vitamin A, such as spinach, oranges, dates and soyabeans.

644 LICK LIQUORICE

Mix ½ teaspoon liquorice root powder with ½ teaspoon honey and ¼ teaspoon clarified butter, then add to 1 cup of milk and take twice daily to help vision stay strong.

645 THORN IN YOUR SIDE

Hawthorn is a great herb for vision as it contains high levels of carotenoids and flavonoids as well as vitamins. Drink a cup of hawthorn tea a day. Alternatively make your own by grinding the dried hawthorn fruits and then infuse in hot water. Strain and mix with honey or maple syrup.

646 PICK PARSLEY

Parsley has long been thought to be a powerful herb to prevent eye problems occurring. Add it raw to food and aim for 25 g (1 oz) each day.

EYE STRAIN

647 TAKE A TEA BREAK

Soak a towel in eyebright tea, then lie down and place it over your eyes for 10 minutes to help get rid of eyestrain. Don't get the tea into your eyes – it's for use as a compress only.

648 CRUSHED MINT COMPRESS

For eye strain, make a cold compress of ice wrapped in a towel or handkerchief. Then crush some mint leaves and place them on top of closed eyes, adding the cold compress on top. Lie still for a few minutes to ease the eyes.

649 COOL AS A CUCUMBER

For a great eye-strain remedy, close your eyes and add slices of fresh cucumber (preferably chilled from the fridge) to the eyelid surface. Relax for several minutes and repeat whenever your eyes feel like they need a rest.

650 PUT A LID ON IT

If your eyelids feel heavy and tired, you can massage a few drops of olive, almond or coconut oil gently along them. Keep the oil and touch very gentle.

PUFFY EYES

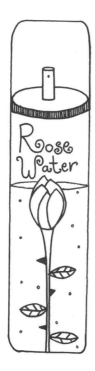

651 BE A ROSE LOVER

Rose water – either the over-the-counter variety or made by steeping crushed rose petals in water overnight – is a great way to reduce baggy eyes as it helps re-moisturize and calm swelling at the same time. Apply using a warm or cold towel depending on which one you find more relaxing.

652 COOL WITH A TEA COMPRESS

Use chilled tea bags, wet and stored for a few hours in the fridge to help them stay really cool and refreshing, as a cold compress to reduce under-eye bagginess. Leave on for 5 to 10 minutes.

653 RAW POTATO TO REDUCE SWELLING

Potato is a great way to help reduce under-eye bags and puffiness. Spritz eyes with water and then apply either thick slices of raw potato or grated raw potato over the eyelids. Leave for 10 minutes.

654 USE A COLD MILK COMPRESS

Soak cotton wool pads in ice-cold milk and apply to your eyes for a few minutes. Re-apply when the compress is no longer cold. Apply for at least 5 minutes and the milk will not only reduce puffiness but is also said to help the whites of your eyes stay white.

655 BEAT PUFFINESS WITH EGG WHITE

To reduce eye puffiness, beat up some egg whites until they are stiff, then add a few drops of astringent witch hazel and mix together. Brush under your eyes to help tighten skin. Leave for 5 minutes before rinsing off with a splash of cold water.

EAR WAX

656 HEAR THE SEA

The best way to remove ear wax naturally is to apply a spritz of salt water in the ear daily. This is a totally safe way to help reduce the build-up of ear wax.

657 OIL IT AWAY

You can use paraffin or any other mineral oil to help reduce ear wax if you have a large build-up. Simply warm a couple of teaspoons of oil on a spoon and drop into the ear, then tip out. Rinsing with a diluted solution of cider vinegar can help restore the natural pH.

658 POUR IN PEROXIDE

For stubborn ear wax, you could try dropping in a few drops of hydrogen peroxide to help dissolve the wax in the ear canal. Make sure you consult your doctor first before doing this.

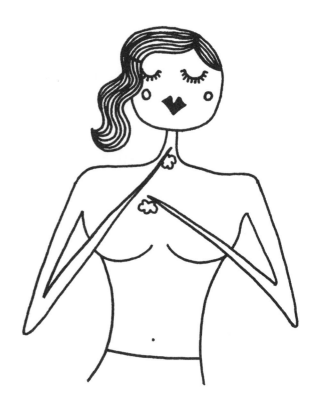

EAR ACHE

659 PLUG WITH COTTON WOOL

Simple cotton wool balls can be used to lessen the pain of earache – gently place a small wad of cotton wool in the outer ear canal (make sure you don't push it down) to help reduce pain. This is especially effective in cold weather.

660 BLOW IT AWAY

One of the best ways to deal with earache is to use your hairdryer to blow warm air into your ear canal. Make sure it is on a low, warm setting and hold it at least 30 cm (12 in) away from the ear.

661 BE A DRIP

A good way to ease middle ear pain (only if your eardrum is not ruptured) is to drip in some warm oil. Warm a little vegetable oil to body temperature, then put a drop or two in your ear canal.

662 INHALE DEEPLY

If you suffer from earache at night it's probably due to blocked eustachian tubes, which don't drain fluids away as efficiently when you're lying down. A great remedy is to perform a decongestant inhalation with eucalyptus oil before bedtime to clear away excess mucus.

663 SEE SESAME

Warm some sesame or linseed oil so it's slightly warmer than body temperature, then add a clove of garlic and allow to infuse for 24 hours. Use a few drops in each ear to help ease earache. Note that you should *never* drop anything into your ears if you think your eardrums might be torn or ruptured.

664 MAKE A LIQUORICE -ROOT POULTICE

For outer ear infections such as swimmer's ear (*Otitis externa*), mix up a paste of clarified butter and liquorice root and spread it around the outer ear. Liquorice has mild antibacterial properties, so is a good way to reduce infections and inflammation.

665 RELY ON RADISH

Make up an ear-calming oil using chopped radish in mustard oil. Store in a glass bottle. If your ear feels sore, a few drops of this warming oil, applied with a dropper, could restore natural balance.

666 PREVENT SWIMMER'S EAR WITH MINERAL OIL

If you are prone to swimmer's ear, you can help prevent the onset by dropping or spraying a couple of drops of mineral oil into your ears before swimming – this helps to dispel the water and avoid infection.

667 A VINEGAR SOLUTION

For instant relief from ear pain, make up a solution of two parts white vinegar and one part alcohol. Use a cotton swab to place a few drops around the outer ear.

TINNITUS & HEARING LOSS

668 STOP INFECTIONS WITH GARLIC

Garlic has long been associated with good hearing, but taking it combined with lecithin in capsule form is also thought to help prevent recurrent ear infections.

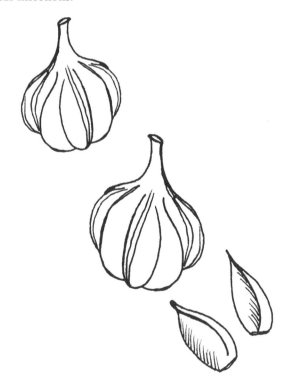

669 GO FOR GINKGO

A few drops of ginkgo biloba liquid extract can be used in each ear to help tinnitus – it's thought that the herb increases blood flow to the ear canal, which can help reduce buzzing and ringing.

670 SALT AWAY THE SOUND

An often-used cure for tinnitus is to wash out the ears with saline water – use freshly salted warm water to wash out both of your ears, leaving the water in your ear canal for a few minutes before draining, if you can.

671 ECHINACEA FOR EARS

Echinacea can be used to aid good hearing equilibrium and reduce dizziness. It also reduces congestion, which can help return hearing to normal. Take in tea or capsule form.

672 TUNE OUT

Most people's tinnitus is worse at night, and if yours follows this pattern and stops you from sleeping, try putting a radio near your bed and tune it between stations to the static noise – this will mask your own ear noises and help you drop off. Ceiling fans or soft music can also work.

YELLOW TEETH

673 BLEACH TEETH WITH PEROXIDE MOUTHWASH

Hydrogen peroxide is safe to use in the mouth, so long as you don't swallow it – simply use as a mouthwash, but make sure you stick to the recommended dilution and amount as it has a strong foaming action. Most home teeth-whitening kits have hydrogen peroxide listed as one of its active ingredients.

674 OIL AWAY STAINS

First, brush your teeth really well to remove all traces of food and plaque. Then, take a clean cloth and dip it in extra virgin olive oil, using it to scrub away at the surface of your tooth. This washes away stains and discolouration and helps your teeth look smooth and white.

675 SALT AND VINEGAR

This is a good remedy for those with badly discoloured teeth, but it shouldn't be done too often as it can be harsh on the tooth enamel. Brush your teeth with salt to help scour off any stains, then dip a toothbrush in vinegar and brush the teeth surfaces – instant results!

676 BAKE 'EM WHITE

Make up a mixture of bicarbonate of soda (baking powder) and water into a paste. Apply to teeth, leave for a few minutes and then rinse and brush normally. You can also use a paste made from bicarb and hydrogen peroxide, if you prefer.

677 REMOVE STAINS WITH SODA

In a bowl, mix 1 teaspoon bicarbonate of soda (baking soda) with a pinch of salt, then add a few drops of white vinegar and mix to a foam. Brush on your teeth before brushing with toothpaste to help remove stains and discolouration.

678 BRUSH WITH COAL

Well, not coal exactly but wood ash from your fireplace – it contains potassium hydroxide, which is a very powerful whitening agent. It doesn't taste good and used regularly could damage your teeth, but if you're after a one-off dramatic chance this could be an option.

679 GO COCONUTS

Using coconut oil as a mouthwash might not seem like a tooth-whitening procedure, but try it every day for a week or so and you'll be amazed at the results.

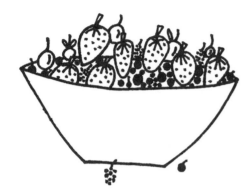

680 SUCK A STRAWBERRY

Strawberries are mildly acidic, which means they can work well as great tooth whiteners. Simply cut a strawberry in half and rub on your teeth, or brush with mashed-up strawberry, leave for 20 minutes and then brush normally. Can be done daily to help keep teeth gleaming.

681 LICK A LEMON

Lemon juice can be used to help whiten teeth, but be careful not to use it too often as the reason why it works is that it robs tooth enamel of calcium. Brush about 20 minutes afterwards, too, to remove sugars.

TOOTHACHE

682 BE A SWEETIE

Vanilla extract rubbed directly onto the gums can help with root pain, like wisdom teeth or teething in infants. Simply use a clean cloth to apply directly to the sore area.

683 POP SOME PEPPERMINT

Peppermint oil is thought to work as a natural painkiller when applied directly to the gum area. It might sting a little on application, but after a few minutes, pain should begin to reduce.

684 USE TOOTHPASTE

For direct toothache, rinse your mouth out with warm water and then apply a dollop of (sensitive) toothpaste directly to the painful tooth cavity. Let it sit for a few minutes before rinsing and try to avoid drinking too much.

685 ALL FOR ALMOND

Almond extract is a great toothache reliever because of its high alcohol content, which dries out the cavity and acts as a topical anaesthetic. Use a few drops on the painful area as needed.

686 OH, FOR OREGANO

You can use oregano to help reduce tooth pain, either by putting dried oregano flakes directly onto the tooth cavity or by making up a mouthwash of warm water, salt and oregano.

687 CHEW ON CATNIP

Catnip is a common garden herb, which is thought to have painkilling properties. Simply chew fresh leaves in the affected area of the mouth to help your toothache reduce in severity.

688 CLOVE THE CAVITY

If you can reach the painful tooth cavity, try adding a few drops of clove oil onto it, or use cotton soaked in clove oil to pack the cavity. Clove is a natural anaesthetic and antibacterial agent, which means it can help reduce pain and inflammation. You can make your own oil by moistening ½ teaspoon ground cloves with olive oil and dabbing around a mouth or gum sore.

689 SLICE AWAY PAIN

Use a slice of raw onion to help reduce toothache pain – simply hold the onion in your mouth and bite gently down on it to release the juices.

690 COUGH AWAY PAIN

If you've got cough drops in your medicine cabinet, you can use them to make a painkilling mouth rinse. Simply add to some hot water, let them dissolve and use the liquid to wash around the painful tooth.

691 GO CRACKERS

Chew a plain water cracker into a paste and use it to fill the tooth cavity. This works by reducing air flow, which eases pain. You can also bite down on a bit of gauze over the top to help keep the wafer plug in place.

692 GET HERBAL

It is thought that taking a combination of cayenne pepper extract, lobelia, valerian root and wild lettuce can help reduce tooth pain. All of these herbs contain calming properties, which may help reduce the severity of the pain. Make your own toothache-healing tea with ¼ teaspoon of each in a cup of hot water, steep for 5 minutes, then strain and drink.

693 A POULTICE FOR PAIN RELIEF

Mix 2 teaspoons bicarbonate of soda (baking soda) with ½ teaspoon each garlic salt, table salt, black pepper. Add lemon juice to make a paste and apply directly to the tooth to reduce pain significantly.

694 WASH WITH SALT

Make up a saltwater rinse with warm water and table salt, and swish it around your mouth, holding it over the affected tooth for as long as you can bear. Spit it out and repeat three or four times.

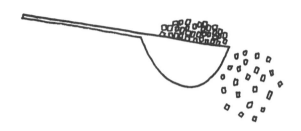

695 USE A TEA BAG COMPRESS

Dampen an ordinary tea bag with hot water, or heat a damp tea bag in the microwave for 10 seconds until hot to the touch (but not burning). Place directly onto the tooth for instant pain relief.

696 GET GARLICKY

Garlic has natural astringent and antibacterial properties, so if your cavity or tooth is infected it's a great natural remedy. If you can bear the strong taste, chew or mash up a raw garlic clove and apply directly to the affected area to reduce pain and inflammation.

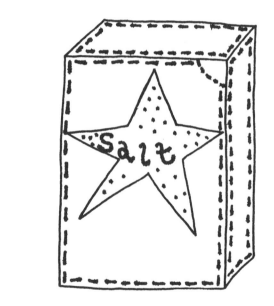

697 GUM IT UP

Get the strongest menthol or peppermint chewing gum you can find (sugar-free), chew it up into a paste and plug it over the tooth area. This helps by introducing peppermint and stopping air from getting to the affected area.

MOUTH & GUM PROBLEMS

698 GET COMFY WITH COMFREY

Regularly taking comfrey and alfalfa is thought to be a good way to prevent tooth decay as both contain high levels of vitamins A, D and C, which are essential for tooth strength. Include these ingredients in your diet.

699 CALL FOR CALENDULA

Calendula and echinacea are both thought to soothe swollen gums and reduce inflammation around gum disease and toothache. They can also be used to treat oral candida infections. Make a strong infusion with a handful of the fresh leaves to 2 cups hot water, then strain and use to swill around the mouth.

700 APPLY LAVENDER OIL

A few drops of lavender essential oil are good for reducing inflammation and protecting against infection; they may also be used to treat candida infections. Apply directly to the affected area. Rosemary oil can also be used in the same way to help treat mouth ulcers and reduce inflammation.

701 HOME-CURE TOOTHPASTE

Make up your own toothpaste using ½ teaspoon salt, 1 teaspoon bicarbonate of soda (baking soda) and a few drops glycerine. The beauty of making your own paste is that you can add your own essential oils to keep your mouth really fresh – try 1 to 2 drops peppermint, spearmint, rosemary or lavender oil.

702 SWISH WITH CRANBERRY

Just as cranberry juice may help to ward off urinary tract infections, it can also be effective against bacteria in the mouth. Swish and drink once a day to help reduce mouth problems.

703 WASH WITH HENNA

Make a tea with henna leaves by infusing 1 teaspoon of fresh henna leaves in 1 cup hot water. Use as a mouthwash to help reduce inflammation and gum problems. This will not stain the teeth, but do not use regularly.

704 HEAL ULCERS WITH JASMINE TEA

Jasmine has good anti-ulcer properties as it promotes skin healing, and heat is thought to help reduce the pain. Combine the two by sipping jasmine tea infusions to help ulcers heal.

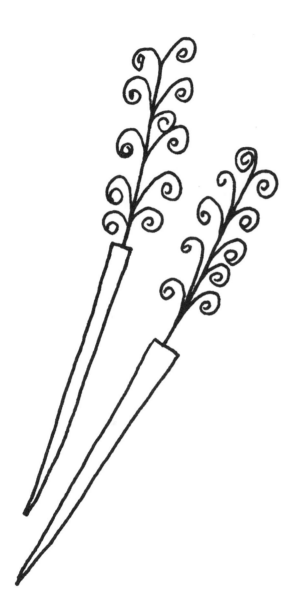

705 CHEW UNRIPE GUAVA

Chewing unripe guava helps stop bleeding and the fruit is rich in vitamin C, which promotes healing. You can also chew the leaves of the guava tree or boil up the bark in water to make a gargle.

706 MAKE A HERBAL MOUTHWASH

Mix 1 teaspoon each dried rosemary, dried mint and fennel seed with 2 to 3 cups boiling water. Allow to steep for 15 to 20 minutes, let cool, cover and store in the refrigerator for 3 to 5 days. Use as a mouthwash to freshen breath and reduce gum problems.

707 IMPROVE GUM HEALTH WITH MUSTARD

Mix 1 tablespoon of mustard oil with 1 teaspoon of table salt. Wash your hands thoroughly and then use a clean finger to apply the mixture to the gums, massaging gently for a few seconds. Rinse well with warm water.

708 CHEW CARROT LEAVES

Keep the leaves from the carrot tops that you usually throw away. Chewing carrot leaves helps mouth ulcers heal more quickly. Rinse well with water afterwards.

709 RELIEVE MOUTH ULCERS WITH TURMERIC

If you suffer from mouth ulcers or sore gums, gargling with plain warm water can help, or make up a mixture of 1 teaspoon of turmeric and ½ teaspoon of rock salt in a large glass of water. This will help reduce inflammation and pain.

710 TRY EUCALYPTUS LEAVES FOR GUM PAIN

Make up a soothing mouthwash for sore gums by boiling a handful of fresh eucalyptus leaves in 1 litre (1¾ pints) of water. Simmer for 5 minutes, then turn off the heat and cover. Strain, add 2 to 3 drops clove oil and bring back to the boil. Allow to cool. Use as a mouthwash after meals and store, covered, in the refrigerator for several days.

711 CHEW A HERBAL TWIG.

Soft neem or acacia sticks (available from Asian and African shops and health food stores) are great natural toothbrushes as they have astringent properties which reduce gum swelling and act as disinfectants. Simply chew on one of these twigs until it softens and splits (usually 5 minutes).

712 RINSE WITH ROSE PETALS

Rose can be both gentle and soothing, reducing inflammation. Boil a handful of rose petals in a small amount of water to extract the essence and mix with a dash of lime, then use as a gargle to soothe sore gums.

713 CALL FOR CITRUS

Lemon, lime and even orange (although it's not quite so potent) are great for helping gums stay healthy as they are acidic and have a high vitamin C content. Rinse with the freshly squeezed juice to help prevent and reduce inflammation of the gums.

714 PASTE A POMEGRANATE.

Dry the rind of a pomegranate and grate it. Heat the grated rind in a little water to make a paste, mashing together. Add salt and pepper. Apply the mixture to the gums for 30 seconds before rinsing to strengthen, stop bleeding and prevent gum disease from developing.

715 PREVENT GUM DISEASE WITH SPINACH AND CARROT JUICE

Spinach juice is thought to act to help prevent gum disease, and its effects are even more potent when taken alongside carrot juice. Combine both in a freshly juiced drink.

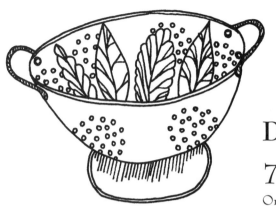

716 CHEW LETTUCE LEAVES

Chewing lettuce leaves immediately after a meal will cleanse the palate and restore the mouth's natural pH values, making gum disease less likely. Keep a few leaves on hand for the end of the meal.

717 FINISH MEALS WITH MINT TEA

Instead of drinking coffee after your next meal, give your mouth a cleanse with a refreshing mint tea. Fresh mint is best, but any infusion will work as peppermint is thought to help teeth and gums remain healthy.

718 FIG-URE IT OUT

Figs are well known in folklore for their ability to help cure mouth sores. Cut a ripe fruit in half and hold it between your cheek and sore gum for 10 minutes to help reduce pain and inflammation.

DENTURES

719 SOAP AWAY BUGS

One of the best ways to keep dentures really clean and free of harmful mouth bacteria is to scrub them with soap and water. As long as you rinse them well afterwards, this is a great way of keeping your new teeth gleaming.

720 ASK FOR ANISEED

Combine 1 teaspoon ground aniseed and 2 teaspoons fresh peppermint in 1 cup boiling water. Allow to cool, then strain and use a couple of tablespoons for rinsing to help reduce the pain of sensitive mouth and gums.

721 SALT OF THE EARTH

When you start wearing dentures or braces, sore spots on your gums can develop quickly. Help keep them from becoming inflamed or infected by rinsing with salt water (½ to 1 teaspoon in a small glass of water) every few hours.

BAD BREATH

722 FIND FENUGREEK

Fenugreek tea is the top home remedy when it comes to clearing up bad breath. Drink the tea several times a day to absorb bad odours and keep breath fresh.

723 CHEW PARSLEY

Parsley is great at getting rid of bad breath – it acts as a natural breath sweetener and deodorizer, which is one of the reasons why it's so often used as a garnish. Chewing parsley after a meal can really help reduce breath odour. Alternatively, steep a handful of parsley in 2 cups boiling water for 5 minutes with a few cloves, strain and use as a mouthwash or gargle.

724 GO FOR GUAVA

Don't wait for that guava in your fruit bowl to ripen – instead, chew on the unripe green flesh to get rid of bad breath in an instant.

725 PICK A POD

After a meal containing strong flavours, if you are worried they may affect your breath, chew a cardamom pod. The flavour is strong but it will neutralize any nasty smells in a few minutes.

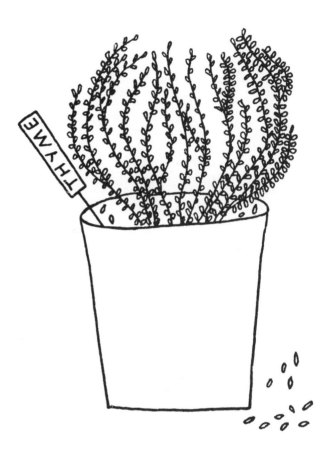

726 MAKE A THYME MOUTHWASH

Pour hot water over a few sprigs of thyme in a cup and steep for 5 minutes, then add a few drops of eucalyptus or tea tree oil. Use as a mouthwash twice a day to help keep breath fresh and clean.

MENSTRUAL PROBLEMS

727 GINGER AWAY PAIN

If you suffer from PMS or menstrual pains, drinking ginger or lemon balm tea can help as they both contain natural analgesics, which help reduce pain and discomfort. Ginger tea is also thought to help make irregular periods more regular, if taken consistently throughout the cycle.

728 CHOOSE VINEGAR

Vinegar is thought to help reduce the pain of menstruation – drink 2 teaspoons apple cider vinegar three times a day, just before meals.

729 MASSAGE PAIN AWAY

Warm a small amount of olive oil (enough to fit into your palm) and rub it onto your lower stomach. Now lie down for 15 minutes and try to relax.

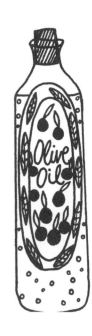

730 REDUCE PAIN WITH CUMIN

If you suffer from severe cramps while you are menstruating, put 2 tablespoons plain yogurt in a bowl and sprinkle over 1 teaspoon cumin and 1 teaspoon honey. Mix well and eat once or twice a day to help ease pain.

731 BUCKWHEAT FOR HEAVY PERIODS

Buckwheat is high in bioflavonoids, which can help reduce bleeding if taken alongside vitamin C. Make a batch of buckwheat pancakes and eat them during your period with vitamin C-rich fruit such as mangoes, raspberries, apples and blueberries. Sprinkle over cinnamon, too, which can help reduce pain.

732 BREW OREGANO TEA

Drinking herbal teas can bring great relief from menstrual pain. Put 1 teaspoon of dried oregano in a cup, pour over boiling water and allow to steep for 5 minutes. Drink slowly, then lie down and rest for the same amount of time it took you to drink the tea. A poultice made with oregano can be used topically to treat menstrual cramps, and camomile and lavender teas are also good alternatives.

733 BATHE IN CAMOMILE

A hot bath is a good way to ease the pain of menstrual cramping – add a cup of camomile tea to the water and put a waterproof pillow under your back, if possible, to take pressure off the lower back and stomach.

734 PASS THE PUMPKIN

Try eating ¼ cup (about a handful) of pumpkin seeds every day for a few days before you get your period to help reduce bloating and discomfort.

735 EAT YOUR BROCCOLI

Broccoli (and fish and beans) are high in potassium, which is thought to help reduce the symptoms of PMS and help the body menstruate without bloating and cramping. Make sure your diet is high in potassium for a few days before you're due.

736 APPLY A HOT COMPRESS

Heat can help reduce pain and cramping, so make yourself a home hot pack to place on your lower stomach. Dampen a face cloth or hand towel, wring out until slightly damp and microwave for 10 to 30 seconds. Test carefully to make sure it won't burn, then relax with the hot cloth placed over your stomach.

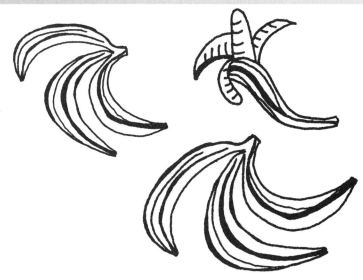

737 GO BANANAS

As soon as you feel the first menstrual cramps starting, eat a banana. Bananas contain high levels of magnesium, which is thought to help relax muscles and lessen cramping, so they're a good choice to reduce pain.

738 THYME FOR BASIL

Basil and thyme are both great herbs to use when you're menstruating as they contain high levels of caffeic acid, known for its pain-killing effects. To brew tea, place ½ teaspoon each dried thyme and basil in a cup, pour over hot water and steep for 5 minutes. Strain and add honey to taste. Drink twice a day.

739 FIX IT WITH FENNEL

Fennel is thought to help reduce cramping during menstruation because it boosts blood flow to the ovaries (incidentally, this also makes it a good choice for boosting fertility in the middle of your cycle). Crush 1 teaspoon fennel seeds in a cup, pour over boiling water, steep for 5 minutes, then strain. Drink three cups a day.

740 DANCE WITH DANDELION

Dandelion root is a powerful diuretic, which can help your body rid itself of excess water and bloating. It also helps regulate the levels of oestrogen in the body, so is good for combating PMS. Capsules, tinctures and teas containing dandelion root can be found in all health food stores. The leaves can be eaten raw in salads and you can make your own coffee – simply dig up a dandelion root (*Taraxacum officinale*) and roast for 10 to 15 minutes, then grind or chop. Steep 1 teaspoon of the root in 1 cup hot water for 10 minutes, strain and drink.

741 RICE IS RIGHT

Rice is a good choice for menstruation as it helps to settle the stomach, reduce pain and alleviate bloating. Choose brown rice and eat once daily.

MENOPAUSE

742 GET WITH THE BEET

When it comes to the menopause, beetroot is one of the best cures. Drink 100 ml (3½ fl oz) of beetroot juice (it's best to juice the vegetables yourself so they're really fresh) twice a day to help relieve symptoms.

743 GET LEVEL WITH LIQUORICE

The symptoms of menopause are caused by differing levels of reproductive hormones. Liquorice can help regulate oestrogen levels, boosting them slightly to reduce symptoms. To make the tea, place ½ to 1 teaspoon licorice root or powder in a cup and pour over boiling water. Allow to steep for 5 minutes, strain and drink three cups a day.

744 HAVE A GOOD EVENING

Evening primrose oil and starflower oil contain gamma linoleic acid, which can help reduce mood swings and breast tenderness. Evening primrose oil is extracted from the seeds of the evening primrose, while starflower is extracted from the herb borage. Take a supplement, but consult your doctor first as they may have interactions with some medications.

745 SAY IT WITH SOYA

Alfalfa, soyabeans, cabbage, sunflower seeds, olives, papaya, oats, peas and sprouts all contain substances which can help stimulate the body's production of oestrogens, reducing the symptoms of menopause. Try to include them in your daily diet.

746 A NATURAL HRT

Consuming 1 teaspoon flaxseed oil twice a day can help mimic the effects of HRT by introducing phytoestrogens to the body, which help reduce menopausal symptoms including hot flushes and vaginal dryness.

747 GET LUBRICATED

If you are suffering from vaginal dryness, make yourself a homemade vaginal cream using 1 tablespoon almond oil and a few drops vitamin E and rose essential oils. Use a clean finger to moisturize the area twice a day.

748 CHOOSE CALENDULA

Calendula is a very mild and moisturizing cream which is a good choice for use as a vaginal moisturizer. Use calendula cream or add calendula essential oil to aqueous cream or almond oil and use twice daily.

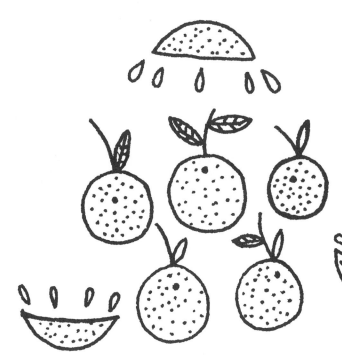

750 SOOTHE DRY SKIN

One of the symptoms of menopause is dry skin. To make your own skin balm mix 1 cup each of beeswax and vegetable oil in a saucepan with a little water. Add the liquid from 1 vitamin E capsule and 2 to 3 drops rose and geranium essential oils. Heat over a very low heat for 30 to 40 minutes. When cooled transfer to a lidded jar; it will keep well for a month.

751 REDUCE HOT FLUSHES WITH SAGE

Sage is a temperature regulator – which is why it's also good for fevers and hot flushes. Add 1 teaspoon dried sage to a cup, pour over boiling water and steep for 5 minutes. Drink several times a day, but allow it to cool down if hot drinks set you off.

749 EAT YOUR PITH

If you're suffering the menopause, make sure you consume high levels of vitamin C and bioflavonoids, which can help reduce symptoms. Also be sure to eat the white pith of citrus fruits and vegetables during this time as this is the part that has the highest concentration. The white pith contains bioflavonoids, such as rutin, which enhance vitamin C absorption.

752 MASSAGE WITH HERBAL OILS

If you suffer from menstrual migraines, use a lavender or rosemary massage oil to massage not only your temples but also the area around your heels at the back of your feet, which can help relieve pain. Or use the herb feverfew (either fresh in salads or in tea) for a stronger painkilling effect.

FEMALE FERTILITY

753 BUY A BANYAN

Banyan (*Ficus benghalensis*) root is available from Asian stores. It can be dried and powdered in a pestle and mortar. Mix 20 g (¾ oz) dried banyan root with 100 ml (3½ fl oz) milk and take before bed for three consecutive nights at the beginning of the cycle, following your period, to help boost natural hormone levels and encourage ovulation. Continue every month until conception occurs.

754 POP YOUR CHERRY

Winter cherry (*Withania somnifera*, also Ashwagandha) is available from health food stores and may help boost fertility. Add 5 g (¼ oz) of the powdered herb to 1 cup milk and drink for five or six nights after menstruation to boost natural hormone levels.

755 EAT AUBERGINE (EGGPLANT)

Aubergine (eggplant) is thought to boost natural hormone levels, which can help increase fertility. Roast aubergine in a medium-hot oven for 20 minutes, then mash with buttermilk to help boost calcium levels at the same time. Eat it for several weeks during your cycle.

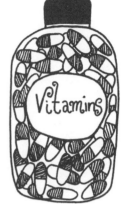
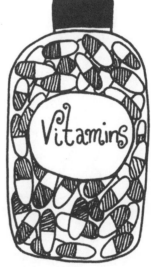

756 BOOST YOUR VITAMINS

If you are having problems conceiving, make sure your vitamin levels are up to scratch. Vitamins C and E are essential for reproductive health because they help lubricate the cervix, while zinc (found in meat, fish and shellfish) promotes proper cell division.

757 BE CAFFEINE-FREE

If you are trying to conceive, swap your usual tea or coffee for naturally caffeine-free green tea or rooibos (redbush), or opt for herbal infusions instead. Caffeine can interfere with fertility.

758 SUPPORT THE SPERM

In order to help the sperm reach the egg naturally, high levels of vitamin C are needed to help lubricate the cervix. Taking grapeseed extract enhances the effect of vitamin C, making the sperm's journey much easier. Place 2 to 3 drops into a glass of water and drink daily; alternatively drink purple grape juice.

759 USE EGG WHITE FOR LUBRICATION

If you need to use a vaginal lubricant for intercourse but you want to conceive, try egg white as it has the least effect on sperm mobility, allowing them to move naturally through the cervix.

760 DOSE WITH COUGH MEDICINE

Taking a dose of cough medicine around the time of ovulation is thought to help boost your chances of conception by increasing the amount of cervical mucus you produce. Take as directed by the manufacturer, and only for two or three nights.

761 FIND FOLIC

Folic acid is essential when it comes to trying to conceive as it is linked to all parts of the reproductive system. Get yours from leafy green vegetables, spinach, orange juice and lentils.

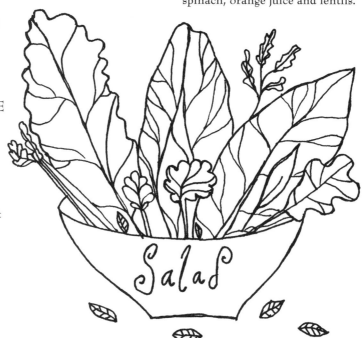

CHLAMYDIA

762 CLEAR CHLAMYDIA WITH SAGE TEA

Sage helps clear your system and speeds recovery from chlamydia – tear and crush a handful of sage leaves and place in a teapot, then pour over boiling water and steep for 5 to 10 minutes. Allow the tea cool, then strain before drinking. Drink 5 to 8 cups throughout the day.

763 CHEW GARLIC

Garlic has strong antibacterial and antiviral properties and helps build immunity – chew on raw pieces of garlic or squeeze to extract the juice and drink 1 teaspoon twice a day while symptoms last.

764 EAT YOGURT

If you have chlamydia, you will probably be prescribed antibiotics. These will get rid of the bacteria, but they may also destroy beneficial bacteria in the body. Eating live (active culture) yogurt can help replace these – take 2 tablespoons three times a day during the course of antibiotics and for three days after the course finishes.

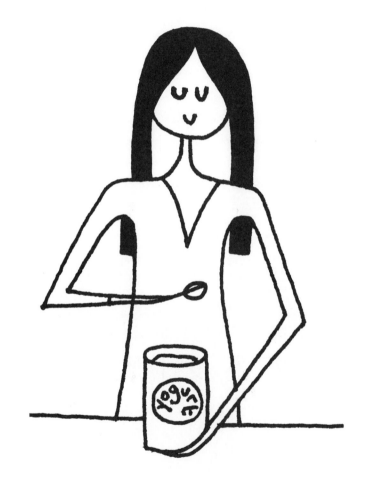

CYSTITIS

765 CURE WITH FRAGRANT JASMINE

Jasmine flowers have been used in Ayurvedic medicine for hundreds of years and are regarded as a sattvic tonic, which encourages the principles of light, harmony and increased perception. Tea made from the flowers reduces fever, treats urinary inflammation and aids the immune system. Jasmine flower compresses made from the cooled tea can also be used to treat heat stroke, headaches or anxiety.

766 COOL AS A CUCUMBER

Cucumber juice is a great choice for combating cystitis as it is a very effective diuretic. To 1 cup cucumber juice add 1 teaspoon honey and 1 tablespoon fresh lime juice. Drink three times a day to help flush away infection. Make sure you stay well-hydrated with water too.

767 CALL FOR COCONUT

Drumstick flowers (*Moringa oleifera*) are available dried or fresh from Asian stores. Mix 1 teaspoon dried drumstick flowers with 120 ml (4 fl oz) coconut water and drink twice daily to help flush cystitis out of your system and reduce pain.

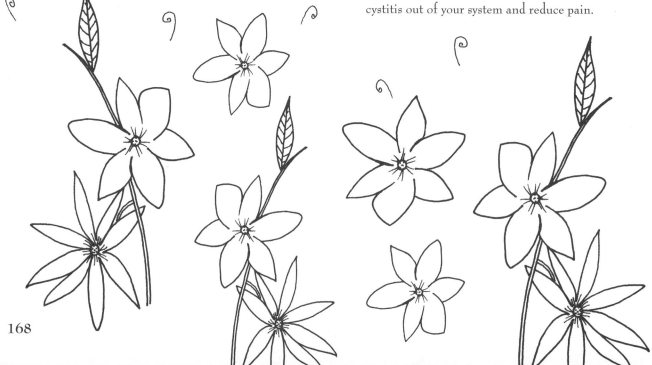

768 CHOOSE CRANBERRY

Cranberry juice is the best-known treatment for urinary infections as it acts as a diuretic, but also coats the inside of the urinary tract to prevent bacteria lodging there and exerts a mild antibacterial effect. Drink a glass a day to help prevent infection or cure cystitis.

769 RISE WITH RADISH

The first thing to do in the morning if you are suffering from cystitis or urinary tract problems is to drink the juice of radish leaves. For best results add them to a juicer or soak overnight and drink the water in the morning.

770 EAT YOUR GREENS

Lady's fingers (okra) and spinach can both be useful against cystitis as they act as very safe, mild diuretics. Eat lightly cooked and pulped for best results.

771 A TEASPOON OF LEMON

Lemon can be used to help treat cystitis because it helps reduce the burning sensation and calms pain and inflammation. Dilute 1 teaspoon lemon juice in 2 tablespoons water and take every few hours while symptoms last.

YEAST INFECTIONS

772 HOME-CURE PESSARY

For a vaginal infection, dip a tampon in plain yogurt containing live cultures of *Lactobacillus acidophilus* and insert into the vagina twice a day until the symptoms clear up. Alternatively, place a few drops of tea tree oil on a tampon and insert into the vagina. Leave for 30 to 60 minutes until symptoms reduce or disappear.

773 DISSOLVE ITCHING

A good way to reduce the itching and soreness of a vaginal yeast infection is to mix 1 tablespoon potassium sorbate (a food preservative available from home-brewing suppliers) in 1 cup water, then soak a tampon in the mixture and insert. Leave for several hours.

774 WASH IT AWAY

Dilute 1 tablespoon apple cider vinegar in 2 cups water and add 1 crushed clove of garlic. Steep for at least 60 minutes, then strain and use as a vaginal wash or douche.

775 FRESH GARLIC CURE

Fresh garlic is great for combating yeast infections – eat a clove once or twice a day at the onset of yeast infection or spread crushed garlic on the affected area and leave for 10 minutes. Garlic paste is a good substitute, but isn't as potent as fresh.

776 MAKE AN ANTI-FUNGAL INFUSION

Licorice, black walnut and goldenseal all have well-known antifungal properties. Take them dried as a tea or used fresh in a cream or ointment.

777 USE A RASPBERRY DOUCHE

Sage and raspberry leaf are both well-known 'women's wellness' herbs. Mix up equal parts of dried sage and raspberry leaf and add one-quarter the amount of dried echinacea. Place 4 tablespoons of the herb mixture in a teapot, pour over boiling water and steep for 15 minutes, then strain and let cool to body temperature. Add 2 tablespoons each cider vinegar and plain yogurt and combine well. Use the mixture to douche every other day (or every day for severe infections) until symptoms disappear.

778 MAKE AN ACIDIC DOUCHE

Acid douches restore the natural pH of the vaginal cavity, which should be quite resistant to yeast growth. Mix 2 to 3 cups water with 2 tablespoons cider vinegar, the juice of ½ lemon or 1 teaspoon liquid vitamin C and douche daily until symptoms disappear.

779 IN-CIDER TRADING

Brush, dab or wash areas affected with apple cider vinegar. If you find vinegar uncomfortable, dilute with water and if your itching is very severe add garlic.

780 CALM ITCHING WITH CAMOMILE

Camomile is a good calming herb to use for the itchiness of yeast infections. Make two cups camomile tea, drink one and use the other to wash the affected area.

781 MILK IT AWAY

The balance of cultures in buttermilk is thought to have a beneficial effect on the body's systems, making yeast infections less likely. Try to include two 250 ml (8 fl oz) glasses a day in your diet.

782 TREAT IT TO A TEA

Tea tree oil, diluted and applied to the area of yeast infection, is a great home remedy for yeast infection as it contains a compound called terpinenol, which is thought to slow yeast growth. Make up a solution with equal parts tea tree oil and surgical spirit (rubbing alcohol) or dilute 4 to 5 drops tea tree oil in 250 ml (8 fl oz) water and use as a douche.

783 DON'T BE A BORE

Boric acid (borax) powder is a great treatment to combat yeast infections. Sprinkle in socks for foot infections, or use mixed with water as a paste for hard-to-cover areas.

784 CHOOSE CRANBERRY

Cranberry juice lowers the pH of your urine, which may be useful in helping to fight off yeast infections by making your whole genital area more acidic. You should choose unsweetened juice as sugar in the diet can actually aid yeast growth.

BREAST SORENESS & BREASTFEEDING

785 CLEAR OUT WITH CAMOMILE

Camomile is a natural diuretic, which can help reduce water retention and bloating. Take as a tea three times a day while you're suffering from breast pain.

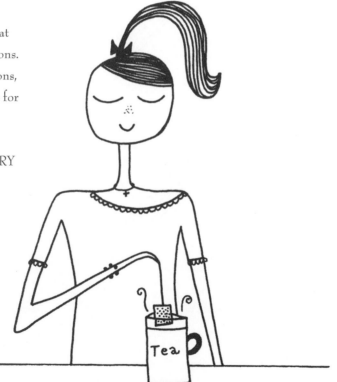

787 DIG DANDELION

Dandelion flowers are a great choice if you have breast pain – they come from the same family as evening primrose but have milder effects. Tear the leaves onto salad or drink as tea to reduce water retention and pain.

788 POP ON SOME ICE

Fill four freezer bags with un-popped corn kernels and freeze them for use as flexible ice packs, which will conform to your breast shape. Ice your breasts after feedings to reduce pain and swelling. When you've finished, simply replace in the freezer to use after the next feed.

789 OPT FOR OLIVE

Olive oil is a great choice for nipple moisturizing if your nipples are feeling sore or cracked because it's totally edible for your baby. Simply apply after feeds and allow to soak into the skin, preferably uncovered.

786 GET FRUITY

Sore breasts are usually due to excess fluid, so choosing foods that can help the body expel water is a good idea – opt for tomatoes, oats, celery, carrots, asparagus and melon.

790 ASK YOUR ELDER

Elder (*Sambucus nigra*) is thought to help reduce breast swelling, particularly if the breasts are engorged. Make an infusion from a handful of fresh elderflowers in 1 cup of hot water. Dip a cloth in the infusion and place on the breast for 5 to 10 minutes.

791 HEAT IT UP

Before feeding, warming the breast can stimulate milk flow, making feeding quicker. Pack a warm towel in a plastic bag and place over the breast for several minutes. This is especially useful if you have sore spots, blocked milk ducts or the beginnings of mastitis.

792 MAKE A CABBAGE-LEAF POULTICE

If you suffer from mastitis, a great cure is boiled cabbage leaves, which help reduce infections in the breast and prevent soreness. Simply cook whole cabbage leaves for 5 to 10 minutes in a small amount of water, then allow to cool until just warm. Place directly onto the breast, holding it in place with a bra for at least 20 minutes.

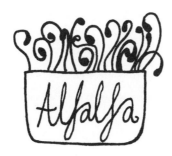

793 CALENDULA CREAM FOR SORE NIPPLES

Calendula is one of the few herbal creams that is safe for baby to swallow, which makes it a good option for applying to cracked and sore nipples – use three or four times a day or whenever the nipples need it.

794 ASK FOR ALFALFA

Alfalfa is thought to help boost milk quality, so it's a good idea to try to include the food in your diet daily. Alternatively, use the herb goat's rue (*Galega officinalis*, available as a powder or tincture), which is thought to boost production by as much as 50%.

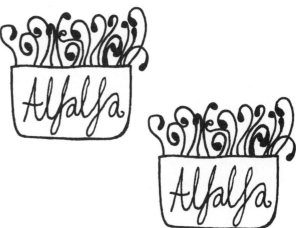

MALE FERTILITY

795 EAT YOUR NUTS

Eating almonds and cashew nuts three times a day will help keep you topped up with all the vitamins you need for excellent sperm health. Eat 5 to 10 nuts each time.

796 ASK FOR ARTICHOKE

Artichoke is a good choice for sperm health as it contains compounds that can help to increase sexual vigour and boost sperm fitness. Eat cooked for best results, with other fertility boosters such as garlic, sardines and celery.

797 GET YOUR OATS

Oatmeal and bran contain high levels of B vitamins, essential for the formation of sperm. Eat them daily for breakfast with raisins, apricot or cherries.

798 HAVE HAWTHORN

Hawthorn is a great choice to keep reproductive organs in tip-top health, especially if you are over 50 years of age. It also helps lower cholesterol and keeps the heart healthy. Try the dried fruits, leaves or flowers as a tea or take as a food supplement.

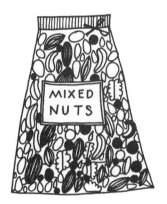

PROSTATE CARE

799 MIX UP AN ALOE CURE

If you suffer prostate problems, mix up a prostate healthy remedy using aloe leaves. Peel 4 aloe leaves and gently cook the whole fibre with 4 tablespoons honey for 15 minutes. Remove from heat, add 3 tablespoons brandy, mix well and drink 1 tablespoon twice a day for a month.

800 SAW IT OFF

Saw palmetto (*Serenoa repens*) is renowned for its anti-cancer properties so it's a great choice to help protect against prostate cancer, especially in people who have family histories of the disease. The berries can be used to make tea, and it is available as an extract.

IMPOTENCE

801 DON'T BE SOFT

Soft-boiled eggs are great for sexual health
as they have high protein levels essential for
strong sperm. For a impotence-beating breakfast,
eat ½ soft-boiled egg with 1 finely diced large
carrot and 1 tablespoon honey. If you suffer
from premature ejaculation, use fresh ginger
root instead of carrot.

802 HAVE A HONEY AND GARLIC INFUSION

Garlic is the most powerful natural remedy against
impotence and it has a clear aphrodisiac effect.
Make an infusion of honey and fresh sliced garlic
root and take 1 teaspoon three times daily before
meals. Alternatively, eat 2 to 3 raw cloves of garlic
a day, spread throughout the day

803 KNOW YOUR ONIONS

Onion increases libido and strengthens the
reproductive organs, particularly if you use
the white variety. Use in cooking every day
or drink a teaspoon of raw onion juice three
times a day.

804 GET HORNY

Horny goat weed (*Epimedium*) is a natural herb that aids circulation and can have dramatic effects on sexual libido and performance. Considered an aphrodisiac in Chinese folklore, it is sold as a health supplement.

805 RAISE THE STAKES

Wash 25 to 50 g (1 to 2 oz) raisins thoroughly in warm water, then boil them with milk until they are swollen and sweet. Drain and eat them, followed by a small glass of the milk, three times a day to help boost sexual health and restore potency.

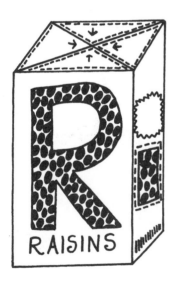

FLATULENCE

806 GO GINGERLY

Mix ½ teaspoon ground ginger with a pinch each of asafetida and salt in 1 cup warm water. Drink when you feel gas or wind pains, but make sure you're in a well-ventilated area as there's only one direction it's going!

807 HAVE A NIGHT-TIME TIPPLE

If you suffer at night-time, add 2 teaspoons brandy to 1 cup of warm water and drink slowly before bed.

808 CHEW GINGER AFTER MEALS

If you suffer from wind after meals, make sure you eat your meals more slowly and give yourself an anti-wind post-prandial by chewing on slices of fresh ginger root soaked in lime juice when you have finished eating. Or add a drop of dill oil to 1 teaspoon of honey and take after your meal for the same effect.

809 REDUCE GAS WITH PEPPERMINT

Chewing peppermint after a meal doesn't just give you fresh breath, it's also good for aiding digestion, including reducing wind, as the menthol soothes digestive muscles. Combine peppermint oil with the same amount of caraway oil to reduce flatulence.

CHILDHOOD TEETHING

810 KEEP COOL

If your child is teething, you can give them relief by providing something cool to bite on. Many babies don't like to bite down on something that is hard, so try keeping a dry cloth in the freezer and giving it to them to bite if teething hurts. Alternatively leave a wet cloth in the fridge for the same results.

811 GIVE BABY A BANANA

Slice several bananas in half and put them in the freezer, then give one to your teething child and allow them to chew on it. The sweetness and coldness will provide relief. Wrap a piece of kitchen paper around the bottom to avoid mess!

812 MAKE AN ICE PACK

To relieve teething pain, wrap an ice cube in a muslin (cheesecloth) cloth, or make a drawstring muslin bag to hold the ice, and give it to your baby to suck – they will enjoy the cool feeling without getting too wet.

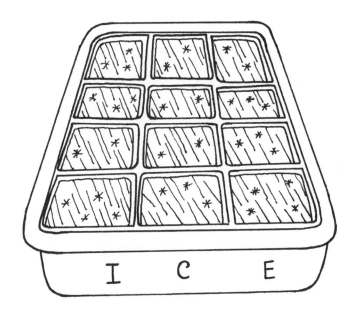

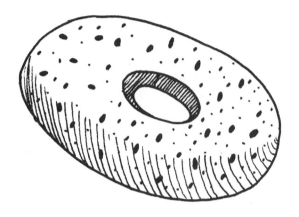

813 BAG A BAGEL

Stick a bagel in the fridge or freezer to create your very own teething ring. It's great for babies to chew on to help teeth cut through the gum and because it's so inexpensive you can replace it easily. You could also try frozen apple or pineapple rings.

814 SPOON IT

Stick a metal spoon in the fridge for a few hours and let your baby chew and suck on it if they are teething to provide relief. The cold metal is a great way to ease gum pain.

CHILD MEDICAL MATTERS

815 THE MAGIC OF MARIGOLD

Very safe for children, marigold can be used in a cream for nappy rash and inflamed and itchy skin, and the cooled tea can be used as rinse for cradle cap.

816 EASE SWELLING WITH CUCUMBER

If your child has swelling anywhere due to illness or injury, simply apply a slice of cucumber to the area. The cucumber has diuretic qualities that will help the body rid itself of fluid.

817 BLOW SOME BUBBLES

Blowing bubbles through a bubble wand can help your child reduce their anxiety levels by forcing them to breathe more slowly. If they seem anxious, get them to blow out slowly to create the longest stream.

818 DAB AWAY FEVER WITH VINEGAR

If your child is suffering from a fever, make up a dilution of equal parts apple cider vinegar and lukewarm water in a bowl. Use a face cloth to dab it on the child's forehead to lower temperature.

819 CARROT JUICE FOR PINWORMS

Grate and extract the juice from 1 carrot (or do this in a juicer, if you have one) and mix with 1 teaspoon honey. Give 1 tablespoon before breakfast and another before bed for three days to help get rid of pinworms.

820 EASE SORE THROAT

If your child has a sore throat, mix together 1 tablespoon each honey and lemon juice, then microwave or heat on the stove. Serve 2 teaspoons of the warmed syrup to ease symptoms (honey should not be given to children under 1 year of age). This can also help croup.

821 ROCK THE CRADLE

For cradle cap, add 3 to 4 drops each eucalyptus oil and lemon oil to 25 ml (1 fl oz) almond oil in a jar. Use a little of the infused oil on your fingertips to massage into the cradle cap and reduce itching.

822 BEAT THE POX

If your child has chicken pox, place 2 to 3 drops camomile and lavender oils in the bath along with 1 cup bicarbonate of soda (baking soda), which will help to heal the skin as they clean and relax your child.

823 VINEGAR FOR CHICKENPOX

Dilute 1 tablespoon apple cider vinegar in 500 ml (1 pint) water. Dab onto the chickenpox lesions to stop them itching and to reduce pain and the chance of infection.

824 VAPORIZE CRYING

If your baby won't stop crying, add a few drops of lavender or camomile oil to a vaporizer in their bedroom and allow the fumes to gently permeate the room. Within a few minutes your baby should feel much more calm. You can also add the oils to a saucer and set down in the bathroom; put the shower on hot for 5 to 10 minutes to create a steam room.

825 MASSAGE AWAY COLIC

If your baby suffers from colic, make a massage oil by adding a few drops of dill or fennel essential oil in 1 tablespoon almond oil. Lie the baby on their back and use the oil to gently massage the stomach and back.

826 FENNEL TEA FOR MOTHER

If your baby suffers colic, what you drink might be able to help if you're breastfeeding. Try cutting back on caffeine and drink fennel tea three times a day.

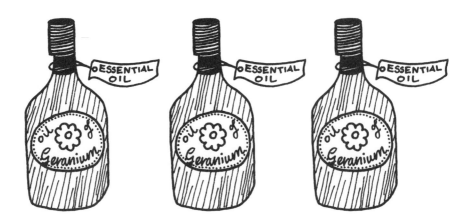

827 ESSENTIAL OILS FOR LICE

To 50 ml (2 fl oz) almond oil add 10 drops each geranium and rosemary oil and 5 drops each lemon and tea tree oil. Massage into the scalp, wrap the head up with a warm dry towel and leave for 2 hours before shampooing out. Comb hair with a fine comb and repeat 48 hours and again one week later to avoid reinfestation.

828 CREATE A SCENTED STEAM ROOM

If your baby has croup, the best remedy of all is steam inhalation. Move them into the bathroom and run the hot water on the bath and shower to create a steam room. Add a handful of the fresh eucalyptus or peppermint leaves, or a few drops of either essential oil, to the water.

NAPPY (DIAPER) RASH

829 SAY IT WITH SESAME

Sesame oil is a good moisturizer for the baby's nappy (diaper) area and it is light enough to be easily absorbed into their skin. Olive oil is another good choice and you can mix either of these with a little water to help thin them out.

830 MIX IN SOME MILK

Breastmilk is sterile as it leaves the body, and is a great moisturizer and skin freshener. Use breastmilk (or regular milk for non-breastfeeders) to massage into your child's bottom to reduce redness and pain.

831 ROAST WHEAT FLOUR

Preheat the oven to 160–180°C (320–365°F).
Pour plain wheat flour into an oven dish and
bake for 10 minutes. Use the baked flour to
spread like talc onto the affected area, reducing
pain and swelling.

832 RINSE IN VINEGAR

If you are using cotton nappies (diapers) rather than
disposables, try rinsing them in a vinegar and water
solution after washing them, making the most of the
antibacterial and antifungal properties of vinegar.
Use the diluted mixture to dab onto nappy rash if
you don't use cotton nappies.

BEDWETTING

833 EAT YOUR NUTS AND RAISINS

Before your child goes to bed (and only if they are
over 5 years old), give them 2 walnut halves and
1 teaspoon raisins to eat. This will reduce anxiety
overnight, which lowers the chances of bedwetting.

834 MASSAGE IT AWAY

Massaging the thighs of your child with St John's
wort oil could help reduce bedwetting by helping
them stay tuned in to signals from the bladder. To
make the massage oil, add 1 to 2 handfuls St John's
wort flowers to a small bottle of a carrier oil, such
as olive or almond oil. Leave in the sun for 2 to 3
weeks, then store in a dark and cool place.

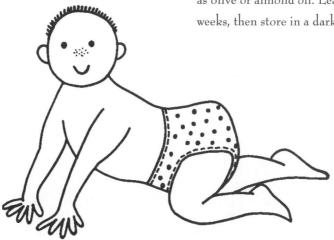

PETS

835 SPRINKLE EUCALYPTUS LEAVES

If you think fleas might be in your home, sprinkle eucalyptus leaves in the places where you think they might be hiding. They don't like the smell, so will move away. You can also rinse their fur with a eucalyptus infusion.

836 SCARE AWAY FLEAS

Make a homemade flea repellant using lemon. Cut a lemon into half and immerse in boiling water, then allow to cool overnight. Strain and use the lemon water to spray all over your pet and their bedding.

837 MASSAGE WITH ESSENTIAL OILS

To remove fleas from fur, make up a mixture of almond carrier oil with a few drops each of lavender and cedarwood oils. Massage through your pet's skin to help keep the fleas away.

838 BATHE IN TEA TREE

If your pet is infested with fleas, you will need to bathe them. Go for total submersion (apart from the head) in a bath containing 3 to 5 drops tea tree or rosemary essential oil.

839 GIVE THEM GARLIC

Give your pet garlic in a little butter, meat or cheese (to entice them). Chop 1 fresh clove of garlic and adding it to 1 teaspoon of the tasty treat, then offer it three times a day. Garlic helps repel fleas because they don't like the taste.

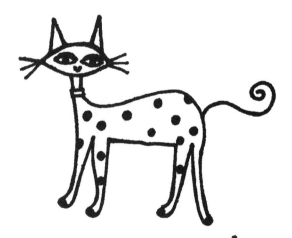

840 BUY THEM A PLANT

Putting a tansy plant (*Tanacetum vulgare*) near your pet's bed is a good way to help repel fleas – make sure you wash all their bedding and blankets regularly too, on a hot wash.

841 GET STINKY

If you want to get rid of skunk odour or other unsavoury smells from your animal, wash their fur in vinegar and water, using rubber gloves to massage it in well. A dilution of hydrogen peroxide and bicarbonate of soda (baking soda) in water may also work.

842 COOL IT AWAY

If your pet has a fever, place a cold compress on their belly (put a tea towel down first), which is one of the best areas for regulating body temperature in animals.

843 CRUNCH CARROTS

If your pet suffers from bad breath, a good way to clean plaque from their teeth naturally is by giving them raw carrots to crunch on.

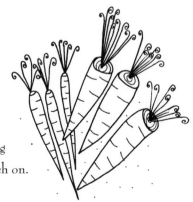

844 LETT-UCE EAT

If your pet has an upset stomach, try to get them to eat some chopped lettuce (mix it with a little of their normal food) as this helps clean through their digestive system.

845 SHAKE OUT EAR MITES

To get rid of ear mites, simply insert 1 to 2 drops mineral oil into your pet's ear and encourage them to shake it out.

846 FEED THEM JUICE

For a urinary infection (more common in cats than dogs) cranberry juice will work just as well for your pet as it does for you. Try to encourage them to drink cranberry juice by soaking a doggie biscuit or animal treat in the juice and offering it to them.

847 PET SMELLS AND SPILLS

For pet spills and urine spots in your house, first wash with warm soapy water, then rinse with clean water and dry. Mix equal parts vinegar and water and dab onto the spot, then rinse and blot dry. Once the area is totally dry (usually 24 hours), sprinkle bicarbonate of soda (baking soda) over the surface and vacuum away.

BOOSTING IMMUNITY

848 GET GREEN AT TEA TIME

Green tea, when taken as a regular part of your diet, has been shown by researchers to be 100 times more powerful as an antioxidant than vitamin C. Drink a warm cup of the naturally low-caffeine green tea twice a day in cold season.

849 ASK FOR ASTRAGALUS

The dried root of the plant astragalus (*Astragalus propinquus*) has long been thought to have immune-boosting properties because of its powerful antioxidant and detoxifying effects, but it shouldn't be taken if you have a fever. Available as a supplement from health food stores, the powdered root can also be made into a tea.

850 FIND A FLAVONOID

To help boost your immunity naturally, try opting for foods rich in flavonoids such as berries, artichokes garlic and yogurt. For a winter boost, freeze berries in the summer when they're cheap and plentiful and mix up yogurt smoothies for a winter breakfast treat.

851 ECHINACEA FOREVER

Echinacea is well known for its immune-boosting properties. Take a daily supplement to help you fight possible infections if you're feeling low or tired, or if you know you're about to be exposed to viruses. If growing at home, wait three years before you use the root; the leaves and flowers can be used sooner. Store the dried root in an airtight tin in a dark place.

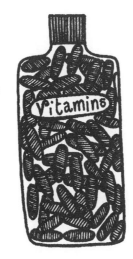

852 C YOUR VITAMINS

The single most important thing for immune boosting is good levels of vitamin C. A person's age and health status can dramatically change their need for the vitamin too. Taking it alongside bioflavonoids can be extra-useful because they aid the body's absorption of the vitamin. Good sources are broccoli, peppers, cauliflower, lemons, greens, brussels sprouts, papaya, cabbage and spinach.

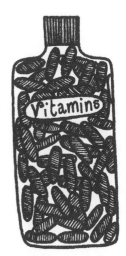

853 BREW UP AN IMMUNE FEAST

To 2 cups of warm water add 1 teaspoon dried and powdered echinacea root and ½ teaspoon each dried camomile and peppermint. Add crushed fresh garlic if you like. Stir well and drink immediately.

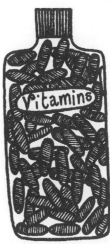

854 JUICE UP A FEAST

Prepare an immune-boosting juice of high antioxidant foods: carrot, beetroot, gooseberries and a pinch of rock salt (with some added fresh garlic), processed in a juicer or liquidizer. The juice has great immune-boosting properties and it doesn't taste quite as strange as it sounds!

855 GO FOR GINSENG

Ginseng, especially Siberian ginseng, when brewed as a tea or used in capsule form, is a great way to help boost your immunity. It is thought to have warming powers as well, so protects against winter colds. If you plan on growing ginseng you need to think ahead: roots take several years to mature but if you plant each year than in two or three years' time you will have a good ongoing supply.

856 REST BETWEEN MEALS

Keeping a proper gap between your meals (not snacking or grazing) is thought to help boost immunity by allowing your body time to reap the full benefits of the food and this will help your energy levels as well.

JETLAG

857 CURB THE CAFFEINE

Some experts suggest using the stimulant caffeine to re-order your body clock. Several days before your flight, start drinking caffeine drinks at the same time of day that you would in the time zone you are travelling to; that way, your body clock will be easier to reset when you arrive.

858 BREAKFAST ON PROTEIN

The day before you fly, start eating high-protein meals for breakfast and lunch and a carbohydrate meal for dinner. Protein in meals stimulates the body to produce catecholamines, which mirrors the body's naturally 'awake' day state.

859 FREE YOUR FEET

Sore feet can be a horrible side effect of flying, but can be relieved with peppermint cream. Add 2 to 3 drops peppermint essential oil to 1 cup aqueous cream. Remove shoes, apply the cream and wear support stocking to avoid puffiness.

860 GO GINGER

If you suffer from motion sickness, take ginger with you on your travels. An acid absorber and blocker of nausea, ginger can be ingested raw, infused, powdered or in capsule form.

861 LICK A LEMON

The next time motion sickness begins to make you feel nauseous, cut a lemon in two and suck on one of the halves. It's thought that lemon can rebalance the acid/alkali balance, which makes you feel sick, so it's worth a try.

862 GET SOME SUN

On the day you are flying, try to get as much sun as possible to help your body's natural melatonin production. That way, you will adjust better to the shifting time zones. Also be sure to get adequate sleep the night before a flight. Called the 'hormone of darkness' melatonin secretion and blood level peaks in the middle of the night, and gradually falls during the second half of the night.

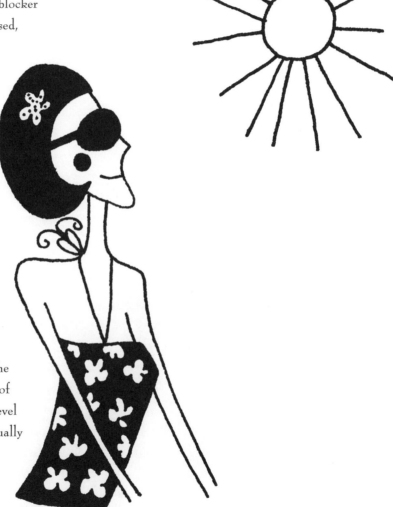

863 RELAX WITH ROSEMARY

The garden herb rosemary is great both for helping relaxation and as an anti-jetlag treatment. Make an infusion from the fresh herb, or add 2 to 3 drops rosemary oil to 1 cup water and drink. Valerian tea can also help you relax and unwind on a flight.

864 EAT OLIVES BEFORE TRAVELLING

It might sound far-fetched, but olives could help reduce motion sickness because they produce tannins, one of the side effects of which is reducing saliva production. Black tea does the same thing, but this will only work if it is taken at the onset of nausea.

865 CRACK OPEN A COLA

Carbonated cola drinks are a great anti-nausea treatment, and they're highly portable, which means they're a great choice to prevent motion sickness. Make sure the drink is carbonated as the air helps calm the stomach by reducing inflammation.

866 WATER IT DOWN

One of the best anti-jetlag treatments is also the cheapest – much of that groggy feeling is actually dehydration, so try to drink a glass of water an hour while in the air to ensure you don't suffer.

TIREDNESS & FATIGUE

867 EAT CRUNCHY SNACKS

If you're tired, you probably feel like reaching for the chocolate for a fast energy boost, but snacking on carrots, celery or cucumber is a great anti-fatigue remedy as they all contain energy-boosting ingredients.

868 SIP UP SOME ENERGY

A great way to boost your energy if you're feeling weary is using citrus fruit juice. It's hard to stay sleepy if you smell lemon, grapefruit or orange. Try juicing your favourite citrus fruits (grapefruit with lemon or lime is a good combination) for an anti-fatigue drink.

869 BRING A BANANA

Potassium is the number one element in combating fatigue, so make sure you are eating lots of potassium-rich foods such as spinach and nuts. Bananas give you lots of easily accessible energy, so try to have one if you are feeling low. Other symptoms of low potassium are cramps, muscle weakness, an irregular heartbeat and dry skin.

870 TIME TO INHALE

For an inhalation to help you beat that nagging tiredness, place some fresh thyme in a bowl and add boiling water. Then cover your head with a towel and breathe in the fumes – it's a great way to give yourself a quick boost.

871 HEAT IT UP

If you're feeling tired, eating spicy food can help, especially 'dry' foods like chilli crackers or fish and meat options such as chilli prawns or beef. Try to avoid creamy sauces and opt for high protein instead.

872 A BASIL AND PEPPERMINT BOOST

Some of the most common garden herbs have great anti-tiredness properties. Try using infusions or tea made with basil and peppermint to give you an afternoon boost.

873 APPLE OF YOUR EYE

Experts don't know if it's the crunchiness, the juiciness or the fact that they're stacked full of healthy nutrients, but apples are the number one anti-fatigue food. Eat the peel too if you can, as the skin contains a lot of the antioxidants.

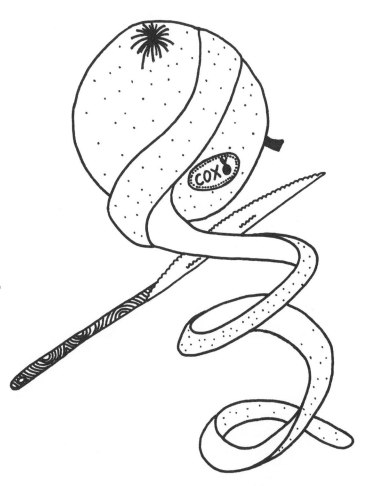

874 RUN A BATH

Having a warm (but not too hot) bath is a good way of reducing tiredness that's due to emotional fatigue. Lavender, clary sage and rosemary are all great herbs to use – just steep them in water or add their essential oils to your bath to help you relax.

875 TAKE A DRINK

One of the major causes of fatigue is being dehydrated. Make sure you drink lots of clear, clean water. Adding some lemon and mint to your water will give you an extra boost.

876 TAKE A SALT BATH

Instead of taking a normal bath if you are feeling tired, use salt water instead. The salt is thought to revitalize you and help your body feel more 'buoyant' even after your bath is finished.

877 PINE FOR PINE

To give yourself a great energy boost for the day, soak a handful of pine needles (collect them yourself) overnight and in the morning, strain and add the liquid to your bath for an instant morning zing. Other evergreen needles will perform the same job.

INSOMNIA

878 CRUNCH A COOKIE

A night-time snack of sugar-laden biscuits (cookies) might not sound like the healthiest choice, but in fact, sugary foods eaten 30 minutes before bedtime can act as a sedative, helping you to drop off to sleep. Stick to one, though – they are high in calories!

879 SNACK ON A SANDWICH

A turkey and lettuce sandwich on wholemeal bread could be the best snack for helping you get off to sleep as it contains high levels of tryptophan, an amino acid that is thought to increase seratonin and thus aid sleep. An hour before bed, eat half a sandwich.

880 CHOOSE VALERIAN

Valerian is a naturally occurring herb that helps induce sound sleep and combat insomnia. Make valerian tea to drink before bed, but be careful to always follow packet instructions regarding dosage and any other medications you are taking. To make your own blend, mix 2 teaspoons each dried valerian root, hops, lemon balm, lavender and camomile. Place 1 teaspoon in a cup and pour over hot water. Allow to steep for 5 to 10 minutes and drink.

881 HIT THE HONEY

Honey is thought to aid sleep because it introduces a complex sugar to the body, which your digestive system can break down easily without strain. Add 1 teaspoon honey to your late-night herbal tea or to warm milk before sleep to ensure you wake rested and relaxed.

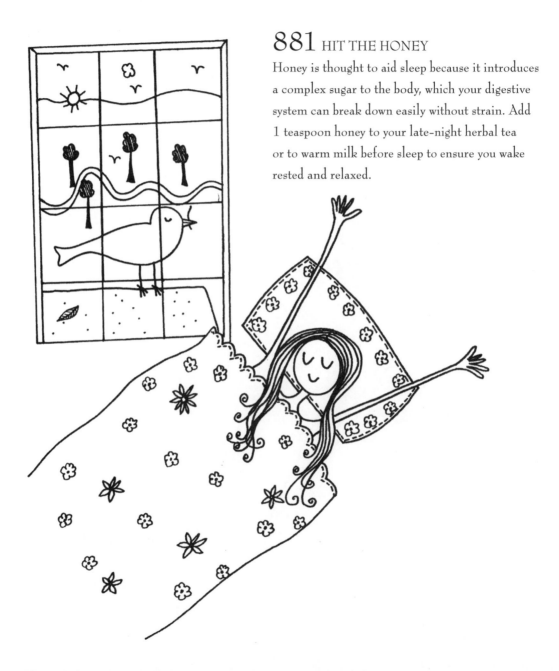

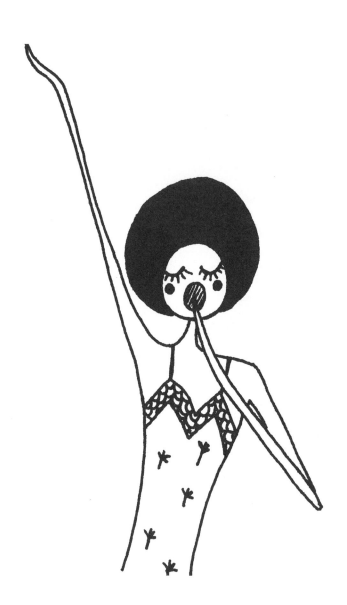

882 SOAK TO SLEEP

Bathing before you retire to bed is a great way to help you drop off to sleep as it helps your body cool naturally. Epsom salts helps your body absorb magnesium, which is essential for calm sleep, so pour a cup into your bath and soak away.

883 CITRUS MAKES YOU SLEEPY

Lemon verbena and lime flower are thought to help induce deep relaxation, which encourages you to fall asleep more quickly and sleep more soundly. Infuse 1 teaspoon of each dried herb in hot water, allow to steep and drink in the evening or before bed.

884 MAKE IT MILKY

A traditional recipe for helping you sleep, warm milk contains not only tryptophan but an opiate-like group of chemicals, which can help you to relax.

885 DRINK SLEEP JUICE

Make up a vitamin-boosting sleep juice. Juice 2 carrots (you could use squash or pumpkin as an alternative), a handful of spinach or lettuce, 2 to 3 dandelion leaves, 3 broccoli flowers and 1 beetroot. Drink 125 ml (4 fl oz) before bed to help you drop off quickly.

886 BATHE IN EUCALYPTUS

Eucalyptus is a great choice for combating insomnia because it helps the body relax, allowing you to drop off more easily. Add 10 drops to an evening bath. The smell also lingers on the skin, continuing to aid calm sleep throughout the night.

887 HOP IT

Hops (*Humulus lupulus*) have a soporific effect, which explains why people who drink beer often feel sleepy. Either buy or harvest the dried strobiles. Before bed add 1 teaspoon dried hops to 1 cup of warm milk, then strain and drink to help you drop off.

888 PAY THE DILL

Dill seeds are thought to have strong sedative effects. Collect seeds after flowering in late spring, then dry in the oven and store airtight container in a cool, dark place. Use dill in your evening meal, to infuse a bedtime drink or in your bath to soak away stress.

889 FILL YOUR PILLOW

Mix together equal amounts of dried peppermint, rosemary, rose, lavender and lemon verbena. Tie up securely in a piece of cotton or muslin and leave in your pillowcase to infuse your sleep.

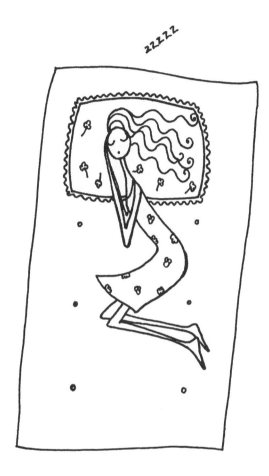

890 BOX IT UP

Next time you finish a box of something like rice or pasta in your cupboard, don't throw away the container – paint it in your favourite colour and turn it into your 'thoughts' box. Keep near your bed with a pad of paper and a pen or pencil. If thoughts or worries keep you awake at night, simply write them down and put them in the box till morning.

891 CALM YOURSELF WITH CAMOMILE

If you believe stress and anxiety is the cause of your insomnia, it's worth drinking camomile tea during the evening. Aim for a cup after your meal and one 30 minutes before bed for best results. Sweeten with honey, if you prefer.

892 GROW LAVENDER INSIDE

Lavender is well known for its relaxing and sleep-inducing effects, but the smell wears off before too long and becomes stale. If lavender helps you, consider growing a lavender plant beside your bed for its natural, full scent and drink lavender tea 20 minutes before you retire.

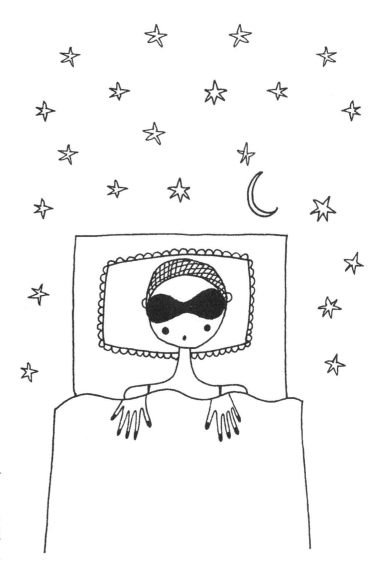

893 RUB YOUR FEET

Rubbing your feet before bedtime for 20 minutes can help reduce stress levels dramatically. Better still, have someone else to do it for you and use your favourite essential oils in a carrier base of olive or sesame oil to help you relax.

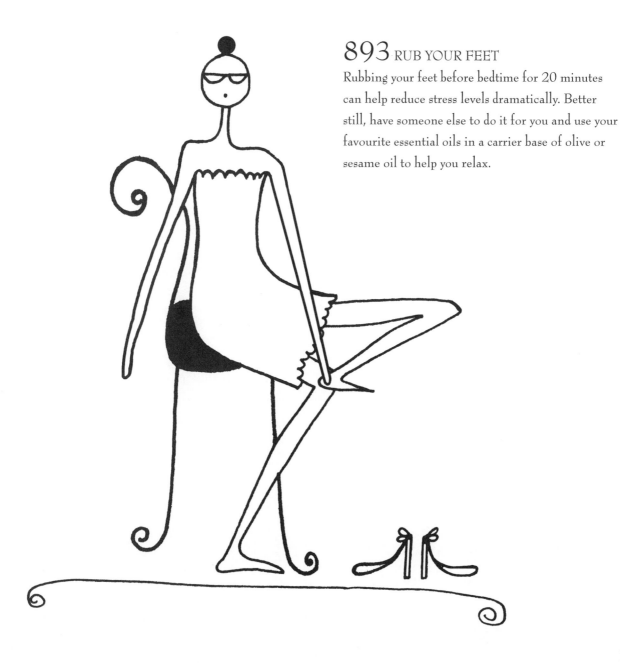

SNORING

894 OIL AWAY SNORING

For a good anti-snore inhalation before bed, rub some Japanese mint oil (available from Asian stores and online) into the back of your hand and inhale deeply for a few minutes before sleeping. It is thought to aid relaxation while tightening the soft palate, so reducing snoring.

895 DON'T BE BITTER

Immature bitter orange (*Citrus aurantium*) has long been used in Traditional Chinese Medicine (TCM) as a snore cure as it contains synephrine, which reduces nasal congestion and allergic reactions. Take the extract under advice from your doctor, though, as it can interact with other medications.

896 PEP UP WITH PEPPERMINT

Drinking alcohol before bed can cause snoring as it relaxes the muscles inside the mouth and throat, and may prevent you waking yourself up to change position. Swap your last drink of the night for a cup of peppermint tea.

897 SPRITZ AWAY SNORING

Make yourself a snore cure by adding 2 to 3 drops peppermint, eucalyptus and olive oils to 1 cup water, adding lemon if desired. Decant to a spray bottle. Use a couple of spritzes on your bedlinen or pillow before bed or during the night to help combat snoring.

898 GARGLE A SAGE INFUSION

Pour boiling water over a handful of fresh sage leaves and allow to cool. Then strain and use to gargle just before bed.

899 PICK SOME PINEAPPLE

Pineapple is thought to help combat snoring problems as it contains an enzyme called bromelain, which reduces inflammation and therefore makes the vibrations that cause snoring less likely to occur. Eat it as an evening snack to help reduce night-time noisiness.

900 BREW UP A SNORE CURE

For a longterm cure to snoring, brew an infusion using 1 teaspoon each dried sage leaves and dried linden flowers in 1 cup boiling water. Allow to cool, strain and drink a cup every day for three weeks in the evening. Linden flowers can be harvested yourself or bought dried from herbal stores.

901 SIP OLIVE OIL

Taking a couple of sips of olive oil before bed is thought to help reduce snoring. Olive oil coats the inside of the mouth, which helps 'trick' the soft palate and throat into feeling 'harder' and thus reducing reverberation. It's also healthy, because it contains essential fatty acids.

902 BE PASSIONATE

For mild snoring, a combination of passionflower and peppermint leaf powder taken as capsules or used to make an infusion has been shown to have some effects. If your snoring is more than mild, add some valerian root powder (but make sure you stick to the recommended amounts).

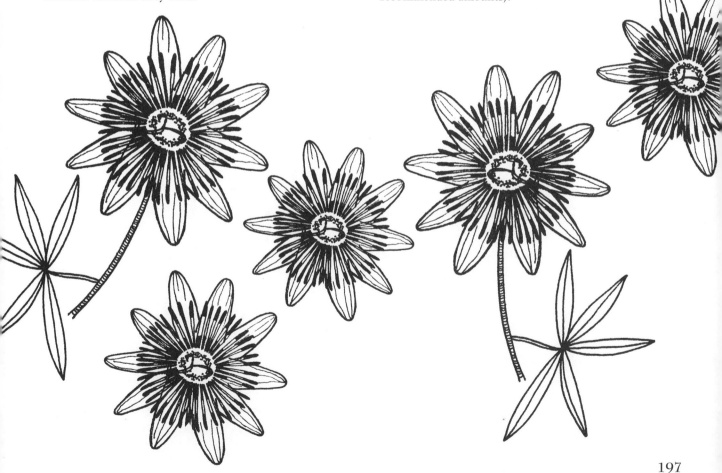

HANGOVER CURES

903 C MORE CLEARLY

One of the best ways to reduce the severity of a
hangover is to consume vitamin C. This means
opting for fresh citrus juice, such as orange or
grapefruit, in large amounts in the morning and
preferably with a glass of water before bed.

904 THYME TO RECOVER

Simmer 6 crushed thyme leaves in 1 cup water
for about 5 minutes. Strain the infusion, allow to
cool, then drink to provide relief from hangovers.

905 GET FRUITY

Hangovers are due to dehydration and toxicity in
the body, so anything with detoxifying properties is a
good choice the morning after. Choose tomato juice,
peppermint, ginger, lemon and cayenne pepper in any
combination you prefer!

906 FLAVOUR WATER WITH LIME

Drinking water is one of the best hangover
remedies as it rehydrates the body and adding
a little lime juice is a great way to boost the taste
and vitamin content.

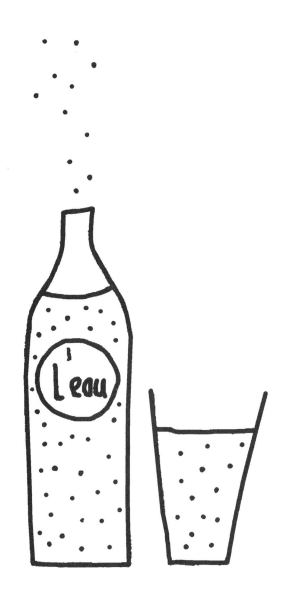

907 BE A HONEY

One of the reasons why people feel bad the morning after drinking alcohol is that the high levels of sugar plays havoc with the body's natural sugar-regulating system. Take 1 tablespoon of honey on waking to help counteract the effects.

908 COAT YOUR STOMACH WITH MILK

After you have been drinking, and before you go to bed, drink a glass of milk. This will help coat your stomach and reduce the toxic effects of the alcohol in your system. Adding chocolate to your milk can also be helpful.

909 LEMON YOUR COFFEE

To help reduce the severity of your hangover, substitute several drops of lemon juice for sugar and milk in your morning coffee and drink slowly.

910 BREW LEMON TEA

A good morning-after drink is unsweetened lemon tea, which will help flush out the toxins from your stomach. The easiest method is to use an ordinary tea bag and add several slices of fresh lemon. Alternatively, mix 2 tablespoons fresh lemon juice in 250 ml (8 fl oz) cold water and drink.

911 CHOOSE COLA

A can of cola is a great morning choice instead of coffee if your hangover makes you feel nauseous. The high levels of caffeine and sugar boost your energy while the bubbles help reduce nausea.

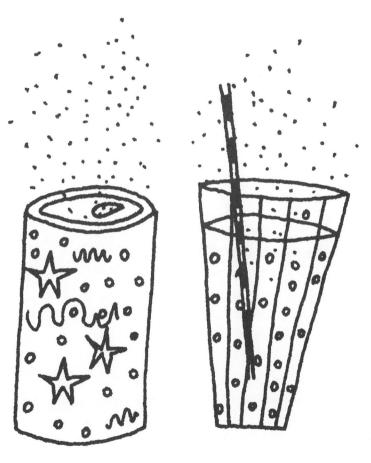

912 SNIFF SOME OILS

Add several drops of peppermint and primrose essential oil to an oil burner, or place in a bowl of hot water. Allow the fumes to permeate the air around you. The fresh clean smells will help your hangover seem much less severe.

913 SOAK A CUBE IN CLOVE

Soak a sugar cube in a few drops of clove oil and suck on it to help reduce hangover severity. Clove has painkilling properties and will help your head feel clearer, while the sugar will replace sugar you have lost overnight as your body metabolized the alcohol.

914 DRY TOAST CURE

Even if you feel really nauseous, you must eat if you want to reduce the effects of your hangover. If you can't face most foods, try dry toast – because the taste is fairly bland, it shouldn't induce sickness.

915 CHEW FEVERFEW

Feverfew is a herb which is thought to help cure headaches and it's a great choice for morning-after headache pain because it has none of the stomach-unsettling side effects of other headache cures. Chew the leaves or brew into a tea.

916 EAT A PRAIRIE DOG

A combination of prairie oyster and hair-of-the-dog, each of the ingredients in this traditional cure has a well-known anti-hangover property. Mix together 1 shot of olive oil, 1 free-range raw egg yolk (unbroken), 1 tablespoon tomato ketchup, a splash each Tabasco, lemon juice and Worcestershire sauce. Add salt and pepper. Drink quickly!

917 TAKE LAVENDER HONEY

Lavender has gentle, calming effects and a great way to benefit if you've got a hangover is to eat 1 teaspoon lavender honey every hour – this will keep your body sugar levels topped up as well as helping you feel calm and relaxed.

918 HAVE A BANANA

In addition to vitamin C, bananas also contain complex sugars which release slowly into the body, providing immediate energy that lasts for several hours. They also contain potassium (which alcohol depletes), magnesium (which can help reduce headaches) and are naturally anti-nauseous.

OVEREATING & OBESITY

919 COOK YOUR CABBAGE

Cabbage contains high levels of tartaric acid, which is why it has long been thought to help weight loss. Substitute one of your meals for a cabbage stir-fry, salad or soup to help reduce your weight naturally.

920 TAKE A TOMATO

Tomatoes fill you up and help balance your body's natural acid–alkali and sugar balance. They also maintain levels of health-giving compounds such as lycopene and antioxidants, which means they are great for weight loss. Try grilled tomatoes at breakfast instead of toast or cereals.

921 GO FOR GINGER TEA

If you find snacking a problem, try switching from coffee or black tea to ginger tea, which can help stave off the desire to snack and boost your metabolism. To make the tea, peel and slice a 2.5 cm (1 in) piece of fresh ginger root and simmer in 4 cups water, covered, for 15 to 20 minutes. Strain, allow to cool and drink.

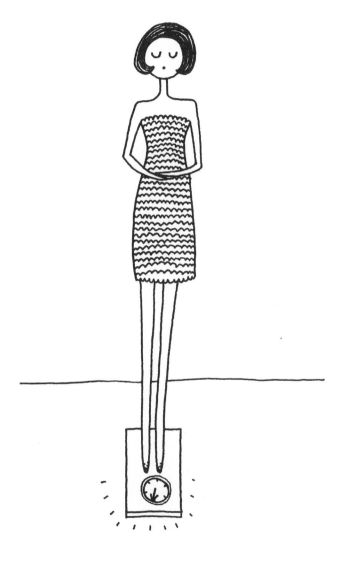

922 CHEW GINGER BEFORE MEALS

To take the edge off hunger, chew a thin slice of fresh ginger root a few minutes before meals. Alternatively, grate a little fresh ginger root, mix with some lemon juice and salt, then eat a pinch or two.

923 GO GREEN

Drinking green tea has been shown to be beneficial in fighting obesity. Choose jasmine green tea or lemon green tea if you find the ordinary type too bitter-tasting, or drink dandelion root tea instead, which has the same effect.

924 DRINK LIME AND HONEY JUICE

Instead of reaching for sugary snacks throughout the day, make yourself a hunger-beating drink by combining the juice of ½ lime with 1 teaspoon fresh honey in 250 ml (8 fl oz) warm water.

925 FINISH WITH MINT

Mint is a good herb to help stimulate weight loss. Add fresh mint to salads and finish off your supper with a peppermint or spearmint tea to aid efficient digestion and beat off late-night snacking. In the summer, keep a jug of iced mint tea in the fridge to drink throughout the day.

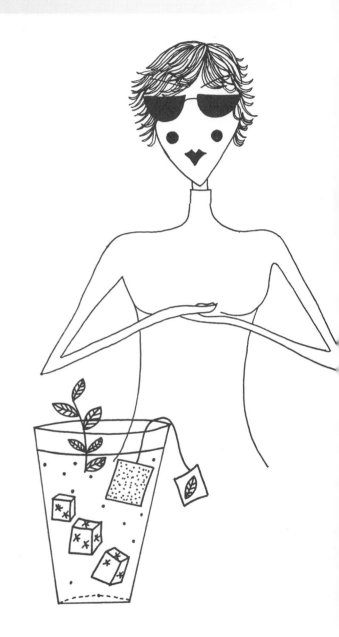

926 DRINK CELERY JUICE

Drinking 150 ml (5 fl oz) of celery juice before each meal will help suppress the appetite. Celery leaves are high in vitamin A, while the stems are an excellent source of vitamins B1, B2, B6 and C, and dense in potassium, folic acid, calcium, magnesium, iron, phosphorus, sodium and essential amino acids.

DEPRESSION

927 BREW BASIL

Drinking basil tea could help you fight off the blues. Put a handful of fresh basil leaves in a teapot and pour over boiling water. Let steep for 10 minutes and drink a cup two to three times during the day to ease depression.

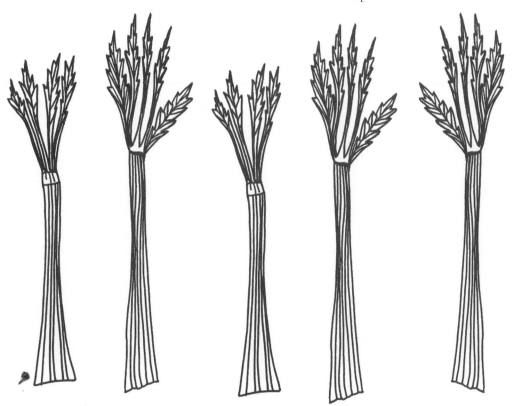

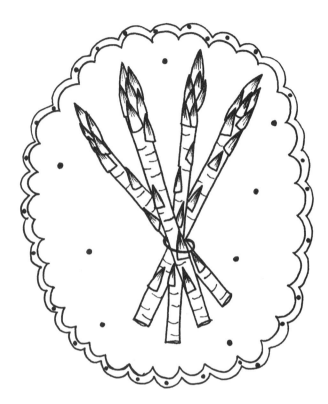

928 ASK FOR ASPARAGUS

Asparagus contains several compounds that can help lift mood and which act as a brain tonic, including folate, which maintains optimal brain function and vitamin E, which is both a mood booster and enhances sexual drive. Eat the stalks fresh, steamed or grilled, or alternatively take 2 grams powdered asparagus root as a depression cure.

929 SMELL GREAT

Make an uplifting refreshing room spray to help boost your mood. Fill a spray bottle with ½ cup distilled water. Then add 12 drops eucalyptus oil, 10 drops lavender oil, 14 drops orange oil and 5 drops tea tree oil. Shake to mix and use as a general room deodorizer.

930 EAT AN APPLE

Experts recommend eating an apple a day as a great way to ward off depression. Apples contain high levels of vitamin B, potassium and phosphorous, which can help your brain repair damaged nerve cells to improve function.

931 CHOOSE CARDAMOM

Cardamom is used in traditional Ayurvedic medicine to improve mood and treat depression. Heat 2 to 3 cardamom seeds in 1 cup of milk, then strain and sweeten with honey, if desired. Drink a glass of cardamom milk a day to help alleviate depression.

932 GET AN AFTER-MEAL SNACK.

After each of your three meals of the day, eat 1 tablespoon honey and 1 raw clove of garlic to help boost your mood.

933 EAT YOUR NUTS

Cashew nuts contain high levels of thiamine, which can help stimulate the nervous system and improve function, plus riboflavin, which can help to improve mood and treat depression. Take a few cashew nuts, raw or slightly warmed, every day.

934 BE CALM WITH CAMOMILE

Camomile tea naturally relaxes the body and mind, reducing anxiety and lifting your mood. Infuse 1 tablespoon fresh camomile flowers in 1 cup boiling water, steep for 10 minutes, then strain and drink. A massage with camomile oil diluted in an almond oil base can also help increase your sense of wellbeing.

935 BOOST YOUR MOOD WITH ROSE

The essential oils present in rose can really help boost your mood, reduce anxiety and fight off rising depression. Place a handful of rose petals, discarding the bitter white bases, in a saucepan. Cover with water and simmer for 5 minutes, then strain and drink 1 cup every day. Alternatively, use rose essential oil to massage your head, face and neck.

936 GO BALMY

Lemon balm is thought to help boost mood if drunk as a cold infusion. To make, soak a handful of fresh lemon balm in a glass of cold water, leave overnight, then strain and drink first thing in the morning for a positive start to the day.

937 LIKE LIQUORICE

Drinking liquorice tea can boost mood and lift depression. Take no more than three cups a day, which otherwise might have adverse effects, and try to space them at regular intervals – morning, noon and night.

938 SOAK YOUR FEET

Soaking your feet in warm water infused with rosemary, lavender or camomile can help you relax. Using either the fresh herbs or essential oils in comfortably warm water, soak feet for about 20 minutes and then pat dry. If you have time, rub on a lavender massage oil to boost the effects.

939 EASE BLACK MOODS WITH SAGE

If taken regularly, sage is a good antidepression cure. Make a tea from fresh sage leaves, include it in stews, soups, risottos and pasta dishes or eat it raw in salads. Include the herb in your diet two to three times a day.

940 SOAK SOME ALMONDS

Almonds are a good choice for beating depression because they contain protein and phenylalanine, which encourages the production of dopamine and noradrenaline. Soak a handful of almonds overnight in milk and eat (with outer skins removed) in the morning before breakfast.

941 BREAKFAST ON OATMEAL

For a good start to the day, make a breakfast with 3 to 4 tablespoons oatmeal in 1 cup rice or soya milk. Add almonds, walnuts, dried fruits like apricots and cherries, and honey. All of these substances have antidepressant properties.

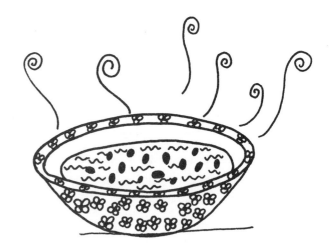

942 LOVE LAVENDER

Lavender tea is another good way to lift mood and induce calm. Place 1 teaspoon dried lavender leaves in a cup, pour over boiling water, steep for 10 minutes, then strain and add honey to taste if desired. Drink three times a day.

943 BE NICE WITH NUTMEG

Add ¼ teaspoon grated nutmeg to 1 teaspoon olive oil, mix well and take three times a day to help lift depression and clear your thoughts.

944 EAT A MOOD-BOOSTING LUNCH

Make a lunch that includes apple, cheese and a glass of water with a spoonful of apple cider vinegar added. All of these contain compounds that can help alleviate the blues.

945 MAKE A MINT AND SPINACH SNACK

Eating 2 to 3 tablespoons cooked spinach with 1 tablespoon chopped fresh mint can help boost your mood. Eat whenever you have a low point during the day, such as mid-afternoon.

946 DRINK A HERBAL WINE TONIC

Add 1 teaspoon dried valerian root (bought or harvested fresh, dried and ground), along with some grated orange peel and a fresh rosemary sprig, to a bottle of white wine. Leave in a cool, dark place for a month, then take 1 tablespoon every day to boost mood. Replace the white wine with vinegar if you prefer not to drink alcohol.

947 AN AVOCADO-LEAF POULTICE

Warm fresh avocado leaves in a small saucepan with 1 tablespoon of water, or microwave for 15 to 30 seconds. Place the warm leaves on the forehead to help alleviate mood. They aid relaxation of the facial muscles, which can lead to a lowering of anxiety.

948 SNACK ON SEEDS

Pumpkin seeds contain high levels of vitamins and minerals, which can help your brain stay positive and healthy, plus having a nutritious snack helps you avoid sugar highs and lows associated with mood swings. Snack on them if you feel your mood lowering.

949 BATHE OUT THE BLUES

A warm bath of slightly salted water can help alleviate depression by relaxing the muscles of the body, back and neck and thus reducing stress and anxiety. Soak for 15 to 20 minutes and follow with a drink of cold iced water with lemon to boost energy.

STRESS

950 SAY IT WITH SUNFLOWERS

Sunflower seeds and alfalfa in combination can help reduce stress by releasing anxiety-lowering substances into the body. Eat them at the very onset of stress to head it off before it begins.

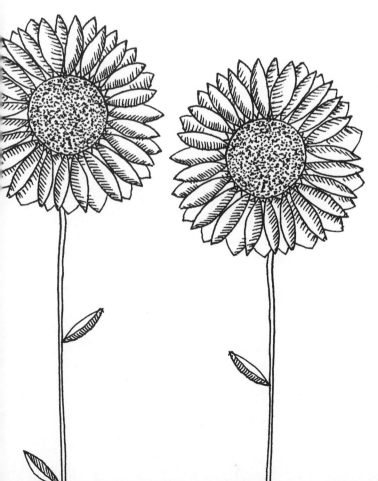

951 SWING FOR ST JOHN

St John's wort is a great herb for beating depression, stress and anxiety. Take it as a tea or powder daily, but be sure to discuss this with your doctor as it can interact with other medications.

952 A SPOONFUL OF YOGURT

Yogurt contains high levels of calcium, vitamin A, vitamin B complex and vitamin D, all of which are linked to relief from insomnia and stress. Take 1 tablespoon three or four times a day to keep your levels topped up.

953 RELAX WITH A GINGER POULTICE

Mix 2 tablespoons powdered ginger with enough milk to form a paste, then apply to the forehead and allow to dry. Your skin will feel slightly warm and then cooler as your facial muscles relax. Leave for 10 to 15 minutes. Wash or wipe off thoroughly.

954 CARRY A HERB POUCH

An idea from the Middle Ages: place ½ cup bishops weed (ajwain) in a muslin (cheesecloth) bag or sachet. Tie with string and carry it around the neck to sniff at the first sign of stress. If you can't find bishop's weed, use rosemary or mint instead.

955 CHUG SOME CHERRIES

Cherries soothe the nervous system, which helps
to relieve stress. Eat them fresh or cooked in pies,
sauces or desserts.

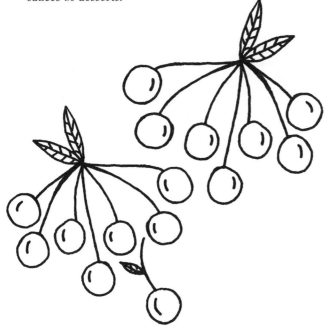

956 BLOW UP A BALLOON

Make yourself a homemade stress ball by filling a
small balloon or sock with rice and gently heating
it in the microwave for 30 seconds in 10-second
bursts. Massage and squeeze the balloon between
your hands for stress relief.

957 CHEW BASIL

If you feel the tides of stress rising, a good anti-stress
treatment for instant relief is to chew a leaf of the
holy basil plant (*Ocimum tenuiflorum*, also known as
tulsi). Simply chew for several minutes to release the
flavours, before swallowing or spitting out. You can
repeat up to 20 times a day with no side effects.

958 BE CALM AT BEDTIME

Bedtime is when stress often rears its head. Beat off
night-time angst with a glass of warm milk flavoured
with cinnamon and honey. If you don't like milk, try
lavender or camomile tea instead.

959 CRUNCH ON CELERY

Celery contains important phytonutrients called
phthalides, which are recognized as sedatives and can
reduce anxiety and stress. Eat celery stalks dipped in
soft cheese or yogurt, or chopped into a salad, once a
day. Lettuce has the same effect.

960 EAT LATE AT NIGHT

Eating late could actually be a good choice for stress
as it helps regulate blood sugar through the night.
Choose pasta, which helps to increase serotonin
levels in the brain.

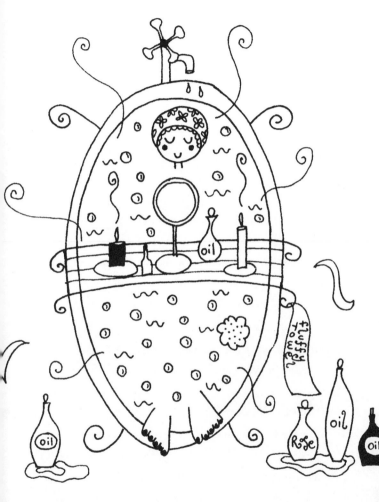

961 A SESAME RUB DOWN

Into a bottle of sesame oil add a few drops of your favourite essential oil, then massage your body all over with the oil before slipping into the bath for a soak. Massage is a great way to help reduce body tension.

962 BATHE IN GINGER

Bathing in a warm bath to which you have added ½ cup each of ginger and bicarbonate of soda (baking soda) can help relieve stress by calming and relaxing muscles that hold tension in the body.

963 HAVE A SALT BATH

Make up a batch of your own bath salts. Mix together 1 cup salt, 2 cups Epsom salts and 4 cups bicarbonate of soda (baking soda). Keep sealed and dry, then add ½ to 1 cup to the bath, along with a few drops of your favourite essential oil, to help soothe away stress.

964 VALERIAN FOR TEA

Valerian is known for its sedative effects so it is a great choice for a bedtime drink to ease away the tensions of the day. Make a valerian tea an hour before bedtime to release stress and anxiety and allow for fresher sleep.

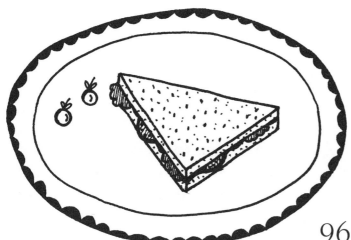

965 GRAB A SANDWICH

Brown bread has high levels of B vitamins, which are thought to sustain the nervous system – try to get about 60% of your daily calories from wholegrains such as wholewheat bread, wholemeal pasta, wholegrain cereal and brown rice.

966 SIP PEPPERMINT

Peppermint tea is well known to relieve tension, but catnip and vervain work well, too. Place 1 teaspoon dried peppermint in a cup, pour over boiling water, let steep for 5 minutes, and then strain and drink before bed. Always take mints with you if you are out (those made with just peppermint and sugar are best).

967 CALM ANXIETY WITH TARRAGON

Tarragon is thought to soothe the nervous system, reducing anxiety, so make a tea by placing ½ teaspoon dried tarragon in a cup, pouring over boiling water, and then steeping for 5 minutes. Strain and drink. You can also add it to salads, soups and stews, or use it as a salad dressing with vinegar or balsamic vinegar and honey.

968 CHOOSE YOUR OIL

Many essential oils have properties which help calm anxiety and tension – try geranium, jasmine, bergamot, neroli, rose, sandalwood and ylang-ylang. Use a few drops in bath water or a foot soak, or add to a carrier oil and use to massage tension points on the body or feet.

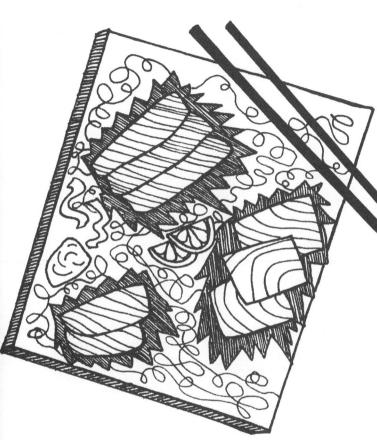

POOR MEMORY

970 PICK A PISTACHIO
Some forms of memory loss may be due to a lack of the substance thiamine, which pistachio nuts contain in very high levels. Just ½ cup contains over one third of your daily allowance.

971 WIN WITH WHEAT GERM
Wheat germ is a great source of vitamin E, which may help with restoring memory, if your memory loss is age-related. Simply add a spoonful to your morning cereal, yogurt or smoothie, or add it to casseroles.

972 GREEN TEA AND PUZZLES
Every day, try to make yourself 1 cup of brain-boosting green tea and sit down for 5 minutes to concentrate on the crossword, Sudoku or other puzzle to give your brain a natural workout.

969 FISH FIRST
Fish oils have been shown to help boost mental health naturally, so make sure you get yours from three to four servings of fish a week, spread across the week. Or take supplements, if you prefer.

973 EXERCISE YOUR MEMORY
The next time you cook a family favourite, do so without using the recipe book. Trying to remember the amounts and writing them down before opening the book could improve your memory.

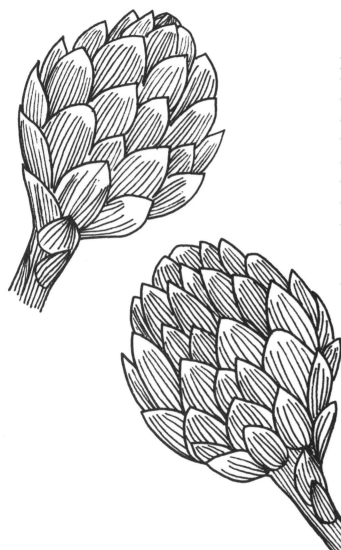

974 DON'T CHOKE

Artichokes are thought to help boost memory and brain function – eat in normal cooking or make an 'artichoke water'. To do this, pull off the leaves and place them in preserving jar. Pour over water to just cover, seal and place the jar in a saucepan of water. Bring to the boil and simmer for 2 hours, then remove the jar and strain the liquid, taking care to squeeze out the contents of the leaves. Take 3 tablespoons three times a day.

975 WORK YOUR LONGTERM MEMORY

You can give your long-term memory a boost just by using your utensils. Ask a family member to take one or two items out of your utensil drawer. The next day have a look and see if you can work out what is missing.

976 TEST YOURSELF

Your memory needs challenges to keep it going. Use your kitchen to help give it a workout. Pick a drawer, open it for 30 seconds while looking inside, then close it and see how many of the contents you can remember. Try to do a different drawer, cupboard or area every day to help keep your brain active.

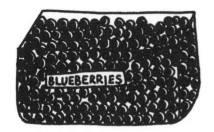

977 GO BLUE

Blueberries are a rich source of antioxidants and vitamins that can help keep your brain in top condition. Eat them raw or cooked every day. Out of season, use frozen blueberries to add to smoothies or desserts.

978 CUT A CARROT

Carrots contain betacarotene, which is a memory booster, and apricots are also a good source. Make up a delicious carrot and apricot juice (using the fresh or dried fruit) and drink every day to help your brain stay flexible and fit.

979 OK FOR OKRA

The combination of minerals and vitamins in lady's fingers (okra) is thought to help prevent memory degeneration and boost brain power. Sweet potatoes and spinach have similar levels, while oranges are another good choice.

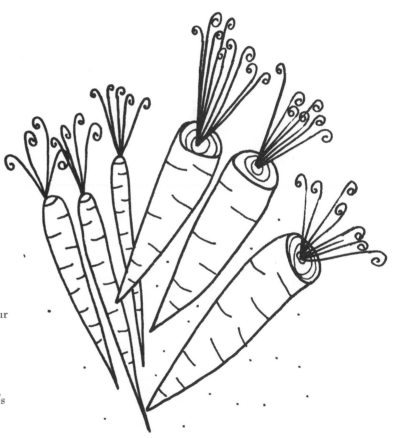

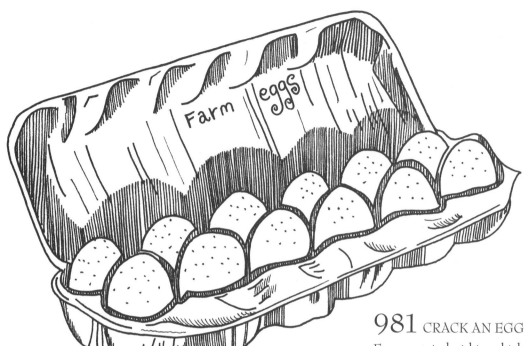

981 CRACK AN EGG

Eggs contain lecithin, which nerve cells (including those in the brain) need to keep them healthy. An egg or two every other day is good, or use sunflower and soya oils, which have lesser amounts of lecithin.

980 TAKE AN INFUSION

Several herbs are thought to help keep your memory sharp if you have a cup of tea made from the infusion of the herb a day. Simply put ½ teaspoon dried basil, sage, rosemary or marjoram in a cup, pour over boiling water, steep for 5 minutes, then strain and drink after breakfast daily.

982 DON'T B A STRANGER

B6 vitamins are widely believed to be the most important when it comes to keeping the memory working well. Also known as pyridoxine, it can be found in cereals, marmite (yeast extract), bread and other complex carbohydrates.

POOR CONCENTRATION

983 HOT ALMOND MILK

Soak 7 almonds overnight in milk, water or orange juice. In the morning, peel and grind into a paste in a mortar and pestle, then mix with a glass of milk. Simmer gently for several minutes and drink while warm. Repeat daily for two to four weeks to help concentration.

984 GO FOR GINKGO

Ginkgo biloba is known to have great memory- and concentration-boosting effects. Try taking it as a supplement.

985 TRY TAURINE IN FISH

If you're looking for a great snack to help you concentrate, choose protein rather than carbohydrates, which can make you sleepy. The amino acid taurine, found in meat and fish, is thought to help boost concentration levels.

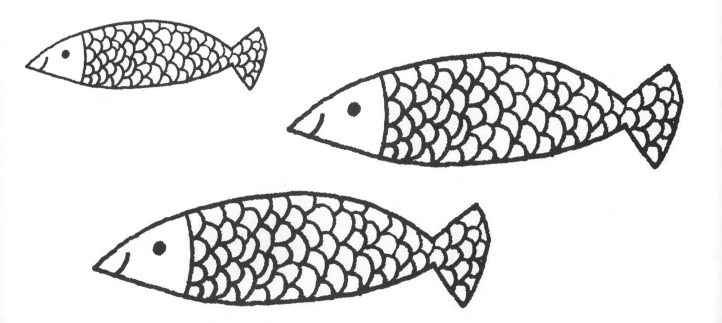

986 GRAB A COFFEE

When it comes to concentration levels, little beats caffeine. A cup of tea or coffee is a great choice to sharpen your brain in the short-term and drink without milk to avoid any soporific effects. Beware of too much, however, as you might end up needing it – stick to 2 to 3 cups a day.

987 GET A GINSENG BOOST

Naturally caffeine-free, a cup of ginseng tea can help boost concentration by focusing energy to your brain, allowing greater focus. Drink for an immediate lift.

988 PRACTISE MAKES PERFECT

Take a candle from your kitchen cupboard and sit in front of it, concentrating on the flame for a minute. Gradually increase the time you spend concentrating on it by 10 seconds a day to help you 'zone in' when you need to.

989 GET A CITRUS BOOST

If you feel your concentration levels flagging, boost them by smelling, drinking or eating citrus fruits, which contain high levels of magnesium. An orange or grapefruit is a good choice to eat, or drink hot water with lemon or lime in the winter. In summer, cold iced water with fruit juice is best.

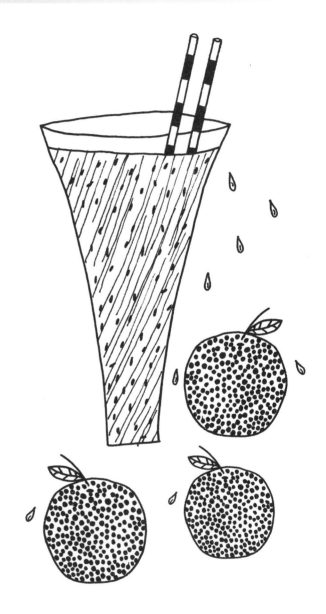

ADDICTIONS

990 STAY RELAXED WITH VALERIAN

Studies have shown that one of the main reasons for giving in to addictions is anxiety – fight yours with valerian tea (the natural source of Valium), which helps detoxify as well as calm nerves and induce calmness.

991 DON'T BE BITTER

Bitter tea, also known as kudzu root, is used in Traditional Chinese Medicine to reduce the appetite for alcohol. It can be bought in health food stores.

992 DON'T B AN ADDICT

Addicts – particularly alcoholics - are commonly deficient in the B vitamins, particularly thiamine. Thiamine is available from quorn, brewer's yeast, pork products, wheatgerm, fish roe and breakfast cereals, so make sure you get the recommended daily amount.

993 SNACK ON MINERALS

Minerals such as calcium and magnesium are most important when it comes to beating addictions physically. Snacking on cheese or yogurt with nuts is the best way to ensure you get both of these in the same meal.

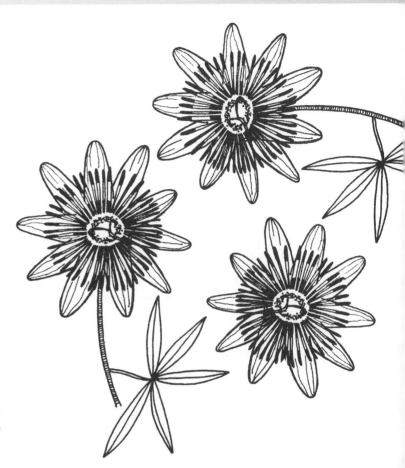

994 GET PASSIONATE

Passionflower is a natural relaxant, which can help reduce anxieties that lead to cravings. It may make you sleepy, so it's a good evening choice – drink as a tea or use as a tincture diluted in water.

995 DETOX WITH DANDELION

Certain plants have natural detoxification properties, such as dandelion, milk thistle and echinacea. Take these regularly as teas or tinctures to help your body recover.

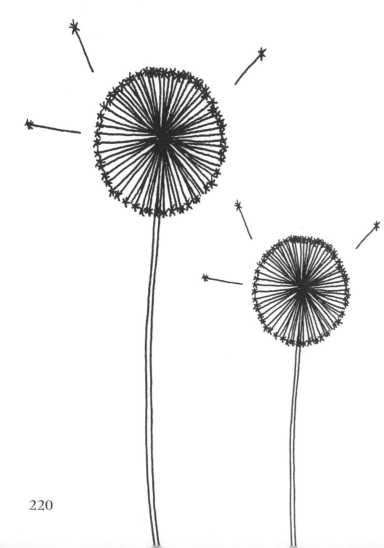

996 REDUCE CRAVINGS WITH SWEETS

One of the best ways to help beat cravings for things like cigarettes and alcohol is to eat something sweet and carbohydrate-filled. This ensures blood-sugar levels are kept high – choose a biscuit (cookie), flapjack or honey-sweetened tea. Grapes are also a good substitution for an alcoholic drink, as they remove toxins from liver.

997 MAKE AN ALCOHOL ANTIDOTE

A great antidote for the toxins present in alcohol is bitter melon juice. Choose unripe fruits (*Momordica charantia*) that are firm, and do not consume more than two gourds a day. It also help cleanse, repair and nourish liver problems due to alcohol consumption. You can mix the juice in a glass of buttermilk and take every morning.

998 STOP ANXIETY WITH SKULLCAP

A powerful medicinal herb, skullcap (*Scutellaria lateriflora*) can help reduce nervous headaches, anxiety and nervousness, especially when combined with heal-all (*Prunella vulgaris*). Add 25 g (1 oz) of the powdered herbs to 500 ml (1 pint) boiling water, steep for 5 to 10 minutes and take ¼ to ½ cup twice a day.

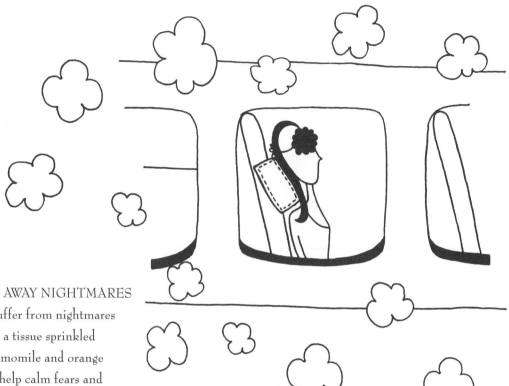

FEARS

999 BREATHE AWAY NIGHTMARES

If you or your child suffer from nightmares or night terrors, leave a tissue sprinkled with a few drops of camomile and orange oil near the pillow to help calm fears and bring sweet dreams.

1000 BEAT VERTIGO WITH GINGER

Try sucking on a piece of crystallized ginger to help allay your fears and dizziness if you suffer from vertigo. The ginger's relaxing and analgesic properties combined with the sugar are thought to help reduce symptoms.

1001 COMBAT FEAR OF FLYING

Herbs that help calm the nerves include St John's wort, skullcap, passionflower and valerian. Dry the herbs and place them in a sachet or small sleep pillow to take onboard.

acacia sticks 157
acid reflux/heartburn 77–8
acne 113–17
addictions 219–20
alcohol 20, 23, 63, 66, 196, 198–200, 219, 220
alfalfa 100, 155, 163, 173, 209
allergies 55–9
almonds 46, 50, 73, 89, 126, 174, 206, 217
  extract 152; leaves 55; oil 9, 47, 51, 124, 134, 146, 163, 179, 181, 182
aloe vera 8, 13, 20, 25, 59, 85, 101, 102, 113, 120, 135, 174
amaranth 72
anaemia 30–31
angina 97
aniseed 72, 158
antiperspirant 19
anxiety 178, 181, 194, 208, 209, 212, 219, 220
apples 30, 33, 48, 62, 77, 84, 110, 116, 126, 189, 204, 208
apricot juice 35, 215
arnica 12, 107
arrack 33
arthritis 98–102
artichokes 90, 174, 184, 214
asafoetida 80, 176
ash-tree leaves 102
asparagus 172, 204
aspirin 15, 35
asthma/breathlessness 68–72
astragalus 184
athlete's foot 142
aubergine (eggplant) 90, 165
avocadoes 104, 133, 208
Ayurvedic medicine 35, 47, 204

back and neck pain 105–7
bacteria, helpful 62, 127, 167
bad breath 159, 183
bagels 178
baking soda see bicarbonate of soda
bananas 49, 68, 95, 104, 110, 122, 131, 162, 177, 188, 200

banyan 165
bark 10, 11
barley 33
basil 8, 33, 34, 42, 49, 59, 69, 87, 97, 162, 189, 203, 216
  holy 31, 69, 71, 210
bath salts 211
bay 132
beans, dried 139
bedwetting 181
bee stings 16
beeswax 14, 164
beetroot 31, 163, 192
bergamot 212
berries 10, 11, 184
bicarbonate of soda (baking soda) 9, 15, 28, 57, 59, 63, 79, 87, 124, 125, 129, 138, 139, 151, 153, 179, 183, 211
bilberries 93
bioflavonoids 164
bishop's weed (ajwain) 209
bites 6, 13–18
bitter melon 220
bitter orange 196
bitter tea (kudzu root) 219
black elder flower 35
black pepper 52, 53, 73, 141, 153
black walnut 65, 170
blackberry leaves 113
blackcurrant 103
blueberries 128, 215
body odour 136–8
boric acid (borax) 171
bran 86, 138, 174
brandy 176
BRAT diet (Bananas, Rice, Apples, Toast) 63
bread 21, 212
breast soreness and breastfeeding 171–3
breathlessness see asthma/breathlessness
brewer's yeast 141
broccoli 109, 161, 192
bronchitis 73
bruises 6, 12, 13, 14, 20
buckwheat 161
bunions 143–4
burns 13, 14, 24–5

bursitis 107
buttermilk 170, 220

cabbage 17, 86, 163, 173, 201
caffeine 19, 70, 86, 166, 179, 186, 199, 218
calamine lotion 18
calcium 104, 110, 111, 203, 209, 219
calendula 23, 96, 155, 163, 173
callouses see corns and calouses
camomile 8, 22, 29, 33, 37, 71, 78, 106, 119, 127, 128, 140, 143, 161, 170, 171, 179, 190, 194, 205, 206, 210, 221
camphor 102
candida infections 155
capsaicin 106
cardamom 31, 34, 159, 204
carpal tunnel syndrome 108
carrier oils 9, 15, 47, 51, 181
carrot juice/carrots 33, 64, 71, 84, 87, 96, 103, 145, 157, 172, 175, 179, 183, 188, 192, 215
carrot leaves 156
cashew nuts 174, 205
castor oil 60
catnip 153
cayenne pepper 8, 36, 44, 88, 107, 141, 153
cedarwood 182
celery 80, 102, 145, 172, 188, 203, 210
cellulite 130
charcoal 18, 62
chasteberry 111
cherries 102, 210
chicken broth 76, 104
chicken pox 179
chicory juice 145
children: bedwetting 181; medical matters 178–80; nappy (diaper) rash 180–81; teething 177–8
chilli peppers 39, 41
chilli powder 105
chlamydia 167
cholesterol, high 89–90

cilantro see coriander
cinnamon 34, 36, 39, 44, 46, 47, 70, 92, 100, 116, 161, 210
circulation 91, 141
clary sage 190
cloves 42, 46, 54, 65, 116, 153, 200
cocoa 74
cocoa butter 119, 127
coconut 65
  milk 65, 118, 134; oil 55, 101, 121, 127, 134, 144, 146, 151; water 168
cod liver oil 103
coffee 19, 29, 70, 130, 199, 218
cola 61, 188, 199
cold sores 18, 59, 60
colds 8, 38, 42–5
colic 179
comfrey 20, 22, 23, 44, 53, 73, 101, 121, 155
compresses, making 11
concentration, poor 217–18
constipation 83–4
COPD (Chronic Obstructive Pulmonary Disease) 73
copper 69, 131
coriander (cilantro) 85, 88, 112
corn kernels 172
cornflour (cornstarch) 60, 124, 126, 142
cornmeal 144
corns and callouses 140–41
cough drops 153
cough medicine 166
coughs 38, 52–4
crackers 82, 153
cradle cap 178, 179
cramps 29
cranberry juice 37, 86, 155, 169, 171, 183
croup 180
cucumber 81, 116, 118, 126, 146, 168, 178, 188
cumin 81, 161
cupboard essentials, top ten 9
cuts 6, 14, 21–3
cystitis 168–9

dandelion 31, 110, 131, 162, 172, 192, 202, 220
dandruff 133–4
decoctions, making 11
dehydration 188, 190, 198
dentures 158
deodorants 137
depression 203–8, 209
dermatitis and rashes 128–9
devil's claw 107
diabetes 92–3
diarrhoea 76
digestion 8, 12
dill 75, 176, 179, 193
dock leaf 18
drumstick flowers 168

ear ache 148–9
ear mites, pets 183
ear wax 148
echinacea 8, 26, 66, 71, 85, 150, 170, 185, 220
eczema 127–8, 129
eggplant see aubergine
eggs 20, 24, 121, 125, 147, 175, 200, 216
elderberries 44
elderflowers 173
elecampane root 71
electrolyte sports drinks 61
emphysema 72
endive juice 145
Epsom salts 9, 27, 60, 83, 96, 104, 129, 132, 133, 140, 144, 192, 211
essential oils 9, 13, 14, 15, 20, 23, 51, 60, 67, 72
eucalyptus 8, 14, 40, 41, 52, 54, 70, 72, 102, 106, 112, 144, 149, 157, 159, 179, 180, 182, 193, 196, 204
evening primrose 163, 200
expectorants 36, 54, 72
eyebright tea 146
eyes: dry 145; eye strain 146; poor vision 145–6; puffy eyes 147

fatigue see tiredness and fatigue
fears 221
feet: athlete's foot 142; bunions 143–4; cold 141;

and colds 45; corns and calluses 140–41; and coughs 52; and headaches 49; reducing a fever 32–5; rubbing 195; smelly 138–9; sore and aching 139–40, 186; toenail fungus 144
fennel 78, 87, 130, 156, 162, 179
fenugreek 44, 71, 93, 120, 134, 159
fertility 165–6, 174
fever 31–5, 178
    pet 183
feverfew 46, 164, 200
fig leaves 66
figs 84, 93, 111, 158
first aid 12–29
fish oils 65, 99, 213
flatulence 176
flavonoids 184
flaxseed oil/flaxseeds 74, 100, 122, 163
fleas, pet 182–3
flowers, drying 10
flu 8
flying, fear of 221
folic acid 166, 203
food intolerances 74
frankincense 23, 73
fructose 94
fruit, harvesting 10

gargles 37, 39, 53, 196
garlic 8, 18, 22, 34, 44, 65, 70, 72, 89, 97, 101, 113, 131, 142, 150, 154, 167, 169, 170, 175, 182, 184, 185
garlic salt 153
geranium oil 130, 164, 180, 212
ginger 8, 22, 34, 35, 37, 39, 42–5, 53, 59, 62, 66, 73, 75, 76, 81, 101, 106, 113, 142, 160, 175, 176, 187, 201, 202, 209, 211, 221
ginkgo biloba 71, 150, 217
ginseng 186, 218
glycerine 121, 124, 137, 155
goat's rue 173
goldenseal 26, 66, 170
gram flour 135

grapefruit/grapefruit oil 35, 37, 41, 79, 130, 142, 166, 188, 218
grapes 33, 41, 54, 79, 90, 122, 220
grazes 6, 13, 14, 21–3
guava 156, 159
gums see mouth and gum problems

haemorrhoids 85
hair: dandruff 133–4; dry hair and scalp 134–5; hair removal 135; thinning hair and hair loss 132–3
hangover cures 198–200
hawthorn 89, 97, 146, 174
hayfever 56, 58
headaches 13, 46–51, 220
headlice 65, 66, 67, 180
heal-all 220
hearing loss 150
heartburn see acid reflux/ heartburn
hempseed oil 128
henna 48, 155
herpes 59–61
hiccups 75–6
high blood pressure 88–9
honey 9, 16, 25, 30, 32, 35, 36, 37, 41, 43, 45, 46, 53, 56, 64, 69, 75, 89, 101, 116, 119, 122, 126, 128, 175, 179, 191, 199, 202, 204, 210
    manuka 9, 59, 117
hops 193
horny goat weed 176
horseradish 32, 107
houseleeks 131
HRT 163
hydrogen peroxide 117, 148, 151, 183

ice 17, 25, 48, 58, 59, 76, 81, 144, 172, 177
ice burn 13, 17, 24, 48
immunity, boosting 184–6
impotence 175–6
incontinence 86
Indian root 71
indigestion 79–80
infusions, making 11

insect bites and stings 15–18
insomnia 190–95, 209
iodine 23
iron 30, 31, 203
irritable bowel syndrome 86–7

Japanese mint oil 196
jasmine oil 212
jasmine tea 155, 168, 202
jaundice 95
jetlag 186–8
juniper 99

karela 94

lady's fingers (okra) 169, 215
lavender 8, 10, 13, 14, 15, 23, 49, 50, 52, 67, 72, 96, 105, 106, 108, 119, 130, 132, 155, 161, 164, 179, 182, 190, 193, 194, 204, 206, 207, 210
lecithin 150
lemon balm 18, 160, 190, 206
lemon juice/lemons 9, 12, 81 acid douches 170; allergies 55; anaemia 30; angina 97; asthma/breathlessness 69; bronchitis/COPD 73; colds 43, 45; concentration 218; corns 141; coughs 52; cystitis 169; dandruff 134; emphysema 72; gums 157; hangover 199; headlice 67; high blood pressure 88; mosquitoes 18; motion sickness 187; nosebleeds 26; rheumatism 103; sore and aching feet 140; sore throat 36, 179; stomach bugs 63; tiredness/fatigue 188; toothache 153; whitening teeth 152; wrinkles 122
lemon verbena 192, 193
lettuce 86, 153, 158, 183, 190, 192
lime flower 192
lime juice/limes 9, 70, 72, 103, 126, 134, 157, 176, 188, 198, 202, 218

linden 33, 35, 196
linseed oil 149
liquorice 73, 146, 149, 163, 170, 206
liver problems 93–4
lobelia 153

magnesium 75, 92, 108, 162, 192, 200, 203, 218, 219
manganese 31
mangoes 36, 84
marigold 21, 49, 178
marjoram 20, 39, 49, 53, 216
marshmallow root 27
mastitis 173
mayonnaise 65, 134
meat tenderizer 17
melatonin 187
melon 47, 80, 88, 172
memory, poor 213–16
menopause 163–4
menstrual problems 160–62
menthol 20, 39, 40, 52, 154
milk: and acne 116; and allergies 56; and asthma 70; bathing in 128; breastmilk 180; and chapped hands 124; and colds 44; and coughs 54; hangover cures 199; and headaches 50; and herpes 60; and insomnia 192, 193; and muscle soreness 104; and osteoporosis 111; and parasites 66; puffy eyes 147; and sore throat 36, 37; and stress 210
milk thistle 93, 220
mineral oil 148, 149
mint 31, 55, 64, 81, 105, 108, 112, 119, 137, 146, 156, 158, 202, 208, 209
miso soup 81
mistletoe 89
moisturizers 28
motion sickness 187
mouth and gum problems 155–8
mouthwash 156, 157, 159
mud packs 127
mullein 69, 71

muscle pain 48
muscle soreness 104–5
mustard 9, 14, 39, 45, 47, 48, 63, 73, 75, 78, 94, 101, 105, 113, 149, 156
    seeds 32, 41, 94
myrrh 85

nappy (diaper) rash 178, 180–81
nasal irrigation 58
nausea 81–2
neck pain see back and neck pain
neem twigs 157
neroli 212
nettles 18, 58, 100, 117
nightmares 221
nosebleeds 26
nutmeg 116, 127, 208

oatcakes 82
oatmeal/oats 9, 28, 41, 86, 90, 113, 123, 126, 138, 163, 172, 174, 206
obesity see overeating and obesity
ointments 14
okra see lady's fingers
olive oil 6, 14, 20, 34, 66, 83, 93, 99, 105, 124, 129, 134, 141, 144, 146, 151, 160, 172, 180, 181, 195, 197, 200
olives 78, 163, 188
onions 16, 24, 35, 36, 52, 53, 70, 72, 85, 91, 97, 118, 140, 153, 175
orange juice/oranges 9, 35, 45, 73, 83, 103, 111, 116, 157, 188, 215, 218
orange oil 204, 221
oregano 93, 153, 161
osteoporosis 108–11
overeating and obesity 201–3

papaya 15, 24, 55, 64, 94, 119, 127, 141, 163
paper cuts 23
paraffin oil 148
parasites 64–7
parsley 38, 45, 80, 81, 88, 92, 97, 145, 146, 159

passionflower 71, 197, 219, 221
pasta 210
patchouli 121
peanut butter 76, 93
peanuts 108
peas 13, 48, 140, 144, 163
pectin 90, 102
peppercorns 33, 69
peppermint 8, 56, 74, 76, 87, 117, 140, 144, 152, 154, 176, 180, 186, 189, 193, 196, 200, 202, 212
peppermint leaf powder 197
peppers 73
pessaries 169
pets 182–3
phosphorus 203, 204
pickle juice 29
pine needles 104, 190
pineapple 39, 79, 110, 141, 196
pinworms 179
pistachio nuts 213
plantain weed 17, 27
plants: harvesting 10; stings 18–19; top ten plants to grow at home 8
PMS *see* menstrual problems
poison ivy 18, 19, 28
pomegranates 33, 64, 157
poppy seeds 55
potassium 95, 110, 129, 131, 161, 188, 200, 203, 204
potatoes 17, 25, 34, 79, 98, 107, 131, 137, 147
poultices, making 11
prairie dog 200
prostate care 174
prunes 83, 84
psoriasis 129
pumpkin seeds 64, 161, 208

quinine 18, 112

radishes 71, 85, 137, 138, 149, 169
raisins 35, 45, 53, 101, 176, 181
rashes *see* dermatitis and rashes
raspberries 52, 82
raspberry leaf 170

rehydration 61, 62, 63, 83, 198
restless legs 112
rheumatism 102–3
rhubarb 90, 102
rice 76, 84, 107, 162
ringworm 66
rooibos (red bush) tea 53
room spray 204
rosacea 120
rose oil/petals/roses 49, 127, 157, 163, 164, 193, 205, 212
rose water 114, 119, 138, 145, 147
rosehip 118
rosemary 47, 48, 66, 67, 91, 96, 104, 132, 156, 164, 180, 188, 190, 193, 206, 208, 209, 216

saffron 35
sage 36, 69, 93, 132, 139, 164, 167, 170, 196, 206, 216
St John's wort 6, 14, 96, 181, 209, 221
salicyclates 35
salt/saline solution 9, 16, 20, 37, 48, 53, 59, 92, 99, 124, 126, 130, 138, 141, 148, 150, 151, 153, 154, 157, 158, 190, 211
sandalwood 46, 55, 119, 127, 212
sardines 74
saw palmetto 174
scars 22, 118–19
seeds, harvesting 10
senna 83
sesame 33, 41, 47, 111, 124, 149, 180, 195, 211
shea butter 127
sinus problems 41–2
skin: dry 123–4; oily 125–6
skullcap 220, 221
slippery elm 27
snoring 196–7
soap 17, 119, 127
sodium 203
sore throats 12, 36–40, 179
soups 43, 44, 45, 81, 100
soya 111

soyabeans 90, 163
sperm mobility 166
spicy food 189
spinach 71, 73, 96, 157, 192, 208, 215
splinters 27
sprains 19–20
sprouts 163
starflower oil 163
stings 6, 13, 14, 15, 16, 17, 18
bee 16, 17; jellyfish 13, 16, 17; plant 18; sea anemone 17
stomach bugs 61–3
strawberries 152
strawberry leaves 113
stress 8, 49, 106, 194, 195, 208, 209–13
stress ball 210
stretchmarks 119–20
sugar 21, 25, 75, 116, 135, 190, 191, 199, 200
sun spots 118–19
sunburn 12, 13, 28
sunflower oil 41, 105
sunflower seeds 163, 209
surgical spirit (rubbing alcohol) 18, 23, 33, 142, 171
sweet potatoes 215
sweets 29, 220
swimmer's ear 149

tamarind 35, 145
tansy 183
tapeworms 66
tarragon 212
taurine 217
tea, making 11
tea tree 9, 13, 19, 23, 40, 41, 59, 60, 67, 117, 129, 131, 137, 139, 142, 159, 169, 171, 204
teeth: childhood teething 177–8; toothache 152–4; yellow 151–2
tendonitis 112–13
thiamine 219
'thoughts' box 194
thyme 33, 56, 70, 130, 159, 162, 189, 198
ticks 66, 67

tinnitus 150
tiredness and fatigue 188–90
toast, dry 200
toddies 43
toenail fungus 144
tofu 111
tomato juice/tomatoes 15, 95, 117, 129, 136, 172, 201
tonic water 18, 112
toothache 18
toothpaste 18, 24, 115, 152, 155
top ten cupboard essentials 11
top ten plants to grow at home 8
Traditional Chinese Medicine (TCM) 196, 219
tryptophan 190, 192
turmeric 21, 44, 53, 68, 113, 135, 157
turnips 136, 139

ulcers 14
urinary infection, pets 183
urine, and sea anemone stings 17

vaginal cream 163
valerian 190, 211, 219, 221
root 153, 197, 208
vanilla extract 152
varicose veins 96
vegetable juices 78
verrucas 131
vertigo 221
Vicks VapoRub 144
vinegar 15, 20, 26, 32, 41, 51, 75, 110, 126, 138, 149, 151, 181, 183
cider 9, 13, 16, 28, 36, 39, 53, 55, 67, 89, 99, 101, 118, 120, 128, 133, 136, 140, 148, 160, 169, 170, 178, 179
vitamins 9, 48, 126
vitamin A 120, 146, 155, 203, 209; vitamin B complex 31, 76, 174, 203, 209, 212, 216, 219; vitamin C 12, 30, 55, 69, 71, 111, 155,

156, 157, 161, 164, 165, 166, 170, 185, 198, 200, 203; vitamin D 155, 209; vitamin E 118, 119, 120, 122, 123, 163, 164, 165, 204, 213; vitamin K (potassium) 21, 31, 109

walnuts 89, 181, 206
warts 131
wasabi 42
water: and acid reflux 77; and hangover 198; and hiccups 76; and irritable bowel syndrome 87
watercress 92
watermelon 47, 88
wheat flour 181
wheat germ 213
wheatgrass 136
white oak 85
white willow/willow bark 35, 46, 107
wine 91, 136, 208
winter cherry 165
witch hazel 14, 85, 96, 114, 121, 129, 147
wood ash 151
wood sorrel 32
worms 64, 65, 66
wounds 12, 22, 23, 27
wrinkles 121–2

yarrow 14, 22
yeast infections 169–71
ylang-ylang 212
yogurt 74, 84, 90, 111, 113, 122, 167, 169, 170, 184, 209
yucca 133

zinc 42, 119, 165

author acknowledgements: Esme would like to thank her mother, Pauline Floyd, for an early education in the importance of remedy-making.